ABC of
Asthma

www.bma.org.uk/library

ABC series

An outstanding collection of resources - written by specialists for non-specialists

The *ABC series* contains a wealth of indispensable resources for GPs, GP registrars, junior doctors, doctors in training and all those in primary care

- **Now fully revised and updated**

- **Highly illustrated, informative and practical source of knowledge**

- **An easy-to-use resource, covering the symptoms, investigations, treatment and management of conditions presenting in your day-to-day practice and patient support**

- **Full colour photographs and illustrations aid diagnosis and patient understanding of a condition**

For more information on all books in the *ABC series*, including links to further information, references and links to the latest official guidelines, please visit:

www.abcbookseries.com

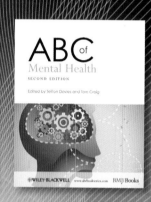

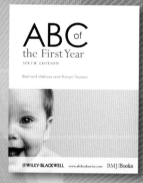

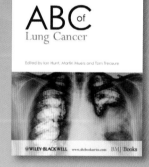

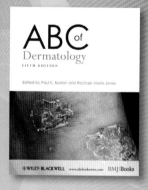

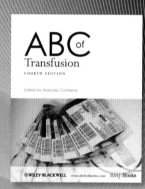

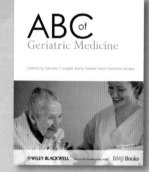

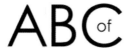

ABC of

Asthma

Sixth Edition

John Rees
Consultant Physician and Professor of Medical Education, Sherman Education Centre, Guy's Hospital, London, UK

Dipak Kanabar
Consultant Paediatrician, Evelina Children's Hospital, Guy's and St Thomas' Hospitals, London, UK

Shriti Pattani
North West London Hospitals Trust, Northwick Park Hosiptal, Harrow, Middlesex, UK
Hatch End Medical Centre, Middlesex, UK

WILEY-BLACKWELL
A John Wiley & Sons, Ltd., Publication

BMJ | Books

This edition first published 2010, © 2010 by John Rees, Dipak Kanabar and Shriti Pattani
Previous editions: 1984, 1989, 1995, 2000, 2006

BMJ Books is an imprint of BMJ Publishing Group Limited, used under licence by Blackwell Publishing which was acquired by John Wiley & Sons in February 2007. Blackwell's publishing programme has been merged with Wiley's global Scientific, Technical and Medical business to form Wiley-Blackwell.

Registered office: John Wiley & Sons Ltd, The Atrium, Southern Gate, Chichester, West Sussex, PO19 8SQ, UK

Editorial offices: 9600 Garsington Road, Oxford, OX4 2DQ, UK
　　　　　　　　　The Atrium, Southern Gate, Chichester, West Sussex, PO19 8SQ, UK
　　　　　　　　　111 River Street, Hoboken, NJ 07030-5774, USA

For details of our global editorial offices, for customer services and for information about how to apply for permission to reuse the copyright material in this book please see our website at www.wiley.com/wiley-blackwell

Library of Congress Cataloging-in-Publication Data

Rees, John, 1949-
　　ABC of asthma / John Rees, Dipak Kanabar, Shriti Pattani. – 6th ed.
　　　　p. ; cm.
　　Includes bibliographical references and index.
　　ISBN 978-1-4051-8596-7
　1.　Asthma.　I. Kanabar, Dipak. II. Pattani, Shriti. III. Title.
　[DNLM: 1.　Asthma.　WF 553 R328a 2010]
　RC591.R43 2006
　616.2′38 – dc22

　　　　　　　　　　　　　　　　　　2009029888

ISBN: 978-1-4051-8596-7

A catalogue record for this book is available from the British Library.

Set in 9.25/12 Minion by Laserwords Private Limited, Chennai, India
Printed in Singapore

1　　2010

Contents

Preface

The prevalence of asthma has increased over the past 20 years and it continues to be a common problem throughout the world. Considerable advances have been made in understanding the genetics, epidemiology and pathophysiology of asthma, new treatments have been devised and older treatments refined.

A small minority of patients have a form of asthma that is very difficult to control but the majority of patients can obtain very good control with standard medications. A number of studies have shown that many patients do not achieve this degree of control. Management of chronic conditions such as asthma is a partnership between patients, families and their doctors and nurses in primary care. This sixth edition of the *ABC of Asthma* deals with recent advances and also contains new chapters that deal with the management of asthma in general practice. We hope that it will help health professionals dealing with asthma and lead to real improvements in the lives of people with asthma.

John Rees
Dipak Kanabar
Shriti Pattani

CHAPTER 1

Definition and Pathology

John Rees

Sherman Education Centre, Guy's Hospital, London, UK

OVERVIEW

- Asthma is an overall descriptive term but there are a number of more or less distinct phenotypes which may have different causes, clinical patterns and responses to treatment
- The clinical characteristic of asthma is airflow obstruction, which can be reversed over short periods of time or with treatment
- In the great majority of asthmatics, treatment is available to suppress asthma symptoms to allow normal activity without significant adverse effects
- Five to ten percent of asthmatics have asthma where control is difficult or side effects of treatment are troublesome
- Inflammation in the airway wall is an important feature of asthma and involves oedema, infiltration with a variety of cells, disruption and detachment of the epithelial layer and mucus gland hypertrophy

---

Asthma is a common condition that has increased in prevalence throughout the world over the last 20 years. It is estimated that around 300 million people are affected across the world. There is no precise, universally agreed definition of asthma (Box 1.1). The descriptive statements that exist include references to the inflammation in the lungs, the increased responsiveness of the airways and the reversibility of the airflow obstruction.

Box 1.1 A definition of asthma

The International Consensus Report on the Diagnosis and Management of Asthma (*Global Strategy for Asthma Management and Prevention*) gives the following definition:

'Asthma is a chronic inflammatory disorder of the airways in which many cells and cellular elements play a role.

The chronic inflammation is associated with airway hyper-responsiveness that leads to recurrent episodes of wheezing, breathlessness, chest tightness, and coughing, particularly at night or in the early morning. These episodes are usually associated with widespread, but variable, airflow obstruction within the lung that is often reversible either spontaneously or with treatment'.

Asthma is an overall descriptive term but there are a number of more or less distinct phenotypes which may have different causes, clinical patterns and responses to treatment.

The clinical picture of asthma in young adults is recognisable and reproducible. The difficulties in precise diagnosis arise in the very young, in older groups and in very mild asthma. Breathlessness from other causes, such as increased tendency towards obesity, may be confused with asthma.

The clinical characteristic of asthma is airflow obstruction, which can be reversed over short periods of time or with treatment. This may be evident from provocation by specific stimuli or from the response to bronchodilators. The airflow obstruction leads to the usual symptoms of shortness of breath. The underlying pathology is inflammatory change in the airway wall, leading to irritability and responsiveness to various stimuli and also to coughing, the other common symptom of asthma. Cough may be the only or first symptom of asthma.

Asthma has commonly been defined on the basis of wide variations in resistance to airflow over short periods of time. More recently, the importance of inflammatory change in the airways has been recognised. There is no universally agreed definition but most contain the elements from the Global Initiative for Asthma.

Low concentrations of non-specific stimuli such as inhaled methacholine and histamine produce airway narrowing. In general, the more severe the asthma, the greater the inflammation and the more the airways react on challenge. Other stimuli such as cold air, exercise and hypotonic solutions can also provoke this increased reactivity. In contrast, it is difficult to induce significant narrowing of the airways with many of these stimuli in healthy people. In some epidemiological studies, increased airway responsiveness is used as part of the definition of asthma. Wheezing during the past 12 months is added to the definition to exclude those who have increased responsiveness but no symptoms.

Airway responsiveness demonstrated in the laboratory is not widely used in the diagnosis of asthma in the United Kingdom but is helpful when the diagnosis is in doubt. The clinical equivalent

ABC of Asthma, 6th edition. By J. Rees, D. Kanabar and S. Pattani. Published 2010 by Blackwell Publishing.

of the increased responsiveness is the development of symptoms in response to dust, smoke, cold air, and exercise; these should be sought in the history.

Labelling

In the past, there was a tendency to use the term *wheezy bronchitis* in children rather than 'asthma' in the belief that this would protect the parents from the label of asthma. More recently, there has been a greater inclination to label and treat mild wheezing or breathlessness as asthma. Self-reported wheezing in the past 12 months is used as the criterion for diagnosing asthma in many epidemiological studies but the symptom of wheezing is not limited to asthma.

These diagnostic trends probably contributed to rising figures on prevalence. However, there were real changes as studies through the 1970s and 1980s also showed increasing emergency room attendance, admission and even mortality. Recent studies show a levelling off or decline in mortality and in asthma attendances in primary and secondary care (Bateman *et al.*, 2008).

The relevance of the early environment has been increasingly evident in epidemiological studies. A significant degree of the future risk of asthma and course of disease seems to be dependent on factors before or shortly after birth (Figure 1.1).

In the great majority of asthmatics, treatment is available to suppress asthma symptoms to allow normal activity without significant adverse effects. These are the goals of most asthma guidelines. However, these treatments are not always delivered efficiently and many patients with milder asthma remain symptomatic (Figure 1.2). Around 5–10% of asthmatics have asthma where control is difficult or side effects of treatment are troublesome. Although we understand more about the onset, pathology and natural history of asthma, little practical advance has yet been made in its cure or prevention.

In infants under the age of 2, wheezing is common because of the small size of the airways. Many of these infants have transient infant wheeze or non-atopic wheezing as toddlers and will not go on to develop asthma. In adults who smoke, asthma may be

THE PREFACE TO THE TREATISE OF THE ASTHMA

SINCE the Cure of the *Asthma* is observed by all Physicians, who have attempted the Eradicating that Chronical Distemper, to be very difficult, and frequently unsuccessful; I may thence infer, That either the true Nature of that Disease is not thoroughly understood by them, or they have not yet found out the Medicines by which the Cure may be effected.

It is my Design in this Treatise, to enquire more particularly into the Nature of this Disease; and, according to that Notion I can give of it, to propose those Methods and Medicines which appear to me most likely to effect its Cure, or, at least, to palliate it.

B

Figure 1.2 The preface to *The Treatise of the Asthma* by J Floyer, published in 1717.

difficult to differentiate from the airway narrowing that is part of chronic bronchitis and emphysema that has been caused by previous cigarette smoking.

Obesity is associated with an increased prevalence of asthma. The associations are complicated with increased airway responsiveness in obesity together with symptoms of breathlessness related to the higher mechanical load on the lungs.

The actual diagnostic label would not matter if appropriate treatment were used. Unfortunately, evidence shows that children and adults who are diagnosed as having asthma are more likely to get appropriate treatment than children with the same symptoms who are given an alternative label. In adults, attempts at bronchodilatation and prophylaxis are more extensive in those who are labelled as asthmatic. Asthma is now such a common and well-publicised condition that the diagnosis tends to cause less upset than it used to. With adequate explanation, most patients and parents will accept it. The correct treatment can then be started. Persistent problems

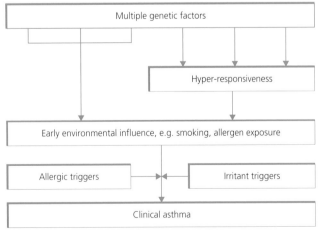

Figure 1.1 Genetics and the environment influence asthma.

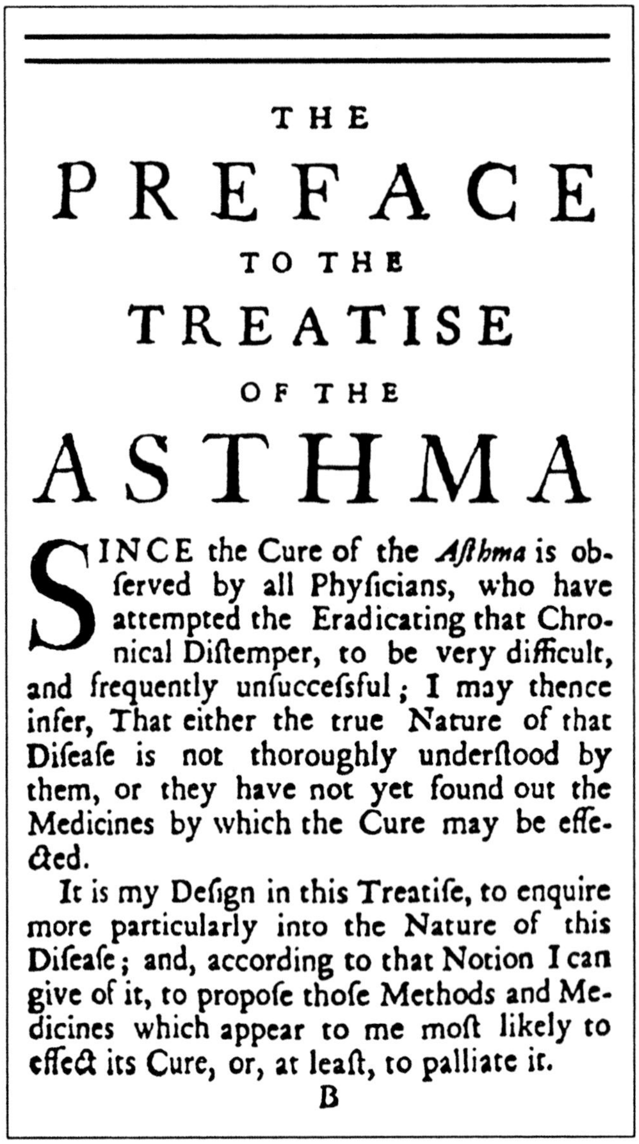

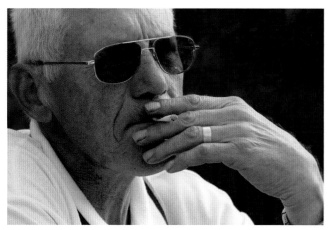

Figure 1.3 In older smokers, COPD may be difficult to distinguish from chronic asthma.

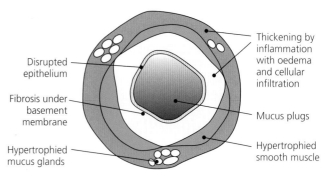

Figure 1.4 Inflammatory changes in the airway.

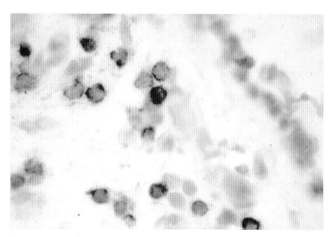

Figure 1.5 CD3$^+$ lymphocytes in mucosa (courtesy of Professor Chris Corrigan).

of cough and wheeze are likely to be much more worrying than the correct diagnosis and improvement in symptoms on treatment. The particular problems of the diagnosis of asthma in very young children are dealt with in Chapter 12.

Treating older patients

In older patients, the commonest dilemma is differentiation (Box 1.2) from chronic obstructive pulmonary disease (COPD) (Figure 1.3). Since both conditions are common, some patients will have both. A degree of increased airway responsiveness is found in COPD in relation to geometry from the narrower airways. Bronchodilators will be appropriate for both conditions although the agent may vary. Inhaled corticosteroids are a mainstay of asthma treatment, when used early, but in COPD, they are less effective and are used to manage more severe disease or frequent exacerbations.

Box 1.2 **Differential diagnosis in adults**	
Chronic obstructive pulmonary disease	May be difficult to differentiate from chronic asthma in older smokers. The pathology differs, as does the degree of steroid responsiveness
Large airway obstruction	Caused by tumours, strictures, foreign bodies. Often misdiagnosed as asthma initially. Differentiated by flow-volume loop
Pulmonary oedema	Once called 'cardiac asthma': may mimic asthma, including the presence of wheezing and worsening at night

Pathology

Since the 1990s, there has been a far greater interest and understanding of inflammation in the asthmatic airway (Figure 1.4). The inflammation in the airway wall involves oedema, infiltration with a variety of cells, disruption and detachment of the epithelial layer, and mucus gland hypertrophy (Figure 1.5). There is thickening of the smooth muscle. Changes occur in the subepithelial layer with the laying down of forms of collagen and other extracellular matrix proteins.

This remodelling of the airway wall in response to persistent inflammation can resolve but may result in permanent fibrotic damage thought to be related to the irreversible airflow obstruction that may develop in poorly controlled asthma.

There is evidence that symptoms in very early life are related to lifelong change in lung function. Very early and prolonged intervention may be necessary to allow normal airway and lung development and prevent permanent changes. In older children, corticosteroids can suppress inflammation, but this returns, with associated hyper-responsiveness, when the drugs are stopped.

The inflammatory cells involved in asthma include eosinophils, mast cells, lymphocytes and neutrophils. Dendritic cells are monocyte-derived cells that present antigen and induce proliferation in naive T cells and primed Th2 cells. The antigen cross links immunoglobulin E (IgE) to produce activation and degranulation of mast cells. T lymphocytes appear to have a controlling influence on the inflammation characteristic of asthma. Th2 lymphocytes that produce interleukin 4, 5, 9 and 13 are increased in the airway in asthma. Inflammatory cells are attracted to the airway by chemokines and then bind to adhesion molecules on the vessel endothelium. From there, they migrate into the local tissue.

In acute inflammatory conditions such as pneumonia, the processes usually resolve. In asthma, chronic inflammation can disrupt the normal repair process; growth factors are produced by inflammatory and tissue cells to produce a remodelling of the airway.

There is proliferation of smooth muscle and blood vessels with fibrosis and thickening of the basement membrane. Hypertrophy and hyperplasia of smooth muscle increase responsiveness which, together with fibrosis, reduces airway calibre. Some of these changes may be reversible but others can lead to permanent damage and reduced reversibility in chronic asthma. A key question is whether early, effective anti-inflammatory treatment can prevent these changes.

The pathological changes may vary between asthmatics, some having predominantly eosinophilic infiltration while others may be mixed or neutrophilic (Anderson *et al.*, 2007).

Clinical evidence

Early evidence on the changes in the airway wall came from a few studies of *post-mortem* material. The understanding advanced with the use of bronchial biopsies taken at bronchoscopy. These studies showed that, even in remission, there is persistent inflammation in the airway wall.

Alveolar lavage samples cells from the alveoli and small airways, giving another measure of airway inflammation. However, it cannot be repeated regularly and is not practical as a monitor in clinical practice. Induced sputum, produced in response to breathing hypertonic saline, is an alternative, more acceptable method which has been used to monitor control.

All these techniques sample different areas and cell populations and by themselves may induce changes that affect repeated studies. However, they have provided valuable information on cellular and mediator changes and the effects of treatment or airway challenge.

A simpler method involves analysis of the expired air. This has been used to measure exhaled nitric oxide produced by nitric oxide synthase, which is increased in the inflamed asthmatic airway. Other possibilities are measurement of pH of the expired breath condensate, carbon monoxide as a sign of oxidative stress or products of arachidonic acid metabolism such as 8-isoprostane. These methods hold promise for simpler methods of measuring airway inflammation but are not in routine use.

Mucus plugging

In severe asthma, there is mucus plugging within the lumen and loss of parts of the surface epithelium. Extensive mucus plugging (Figure 1.6) is the striking finding in the lungs of patients who die of an acute exacerbation of asthma.

Asthma as a general condition

It has been suggested that asthma is a generalised abnormality of the inflammatory or immune cells and that the lungs are just the site where the symptoms show. This does not explain the finding that lungs from a donor with mild asthma transplanted into a non-asthmatic produced problems with obstruction of airflow while normal lungs transplanted into an asthmatic patient were free of problems. However, the link to the nasal mucosa has been recognised more widely. The same trigger factors may affect both

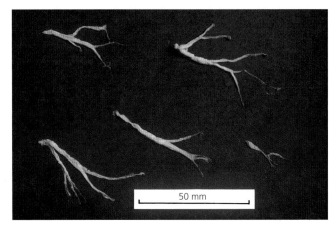

Figure 1.6 Extensive airway plugs and casts of airways can occur in severe asthma (Curschmann's spirals).

areas of the respiratory tract. A combined approach to treatment may be very helpful in control of each area.

Types of asthma

Most asthma develops during childhood and usually varies considerably with time and treatment (Table 1.1). Young asthmatic patients usually have identifiable triggers that provoke wheezing, although there is seldom one single extrinsic cause for all their attacks. This 'extrinsic' asthma is often associated with other features of atopy such as rhinitis and eczema. When asthma starts in adult life, the airflow obstruction is often more persistent and many exacerbations have no obvious stimuli other than respiratory

Table 1.1 Types of asthma.

Childhood onset	Most asthma starts in childhood, usually on an atopic background. Tends to have significant variability and identifiable precipitants
Adult onset	Often a relapse of earlier asthma, but may have initial onset at any age. Often more persistent with fewer obvious precipitants except infection
Nocturnal	Common in all types of asthma, related to poor overall control and increased reactivity
Occupational	Underdiagnosed, needs expert evaluation
Cough-variant	Cough is a common symptom and may precede airflow obstruction
Exercise-induced	Common precipitant, exercise may be the only significant precipitant in children
Brittle	Type 1: chaotic uncontrolled asthma with very variable peak flow
	Type 2: sudden severe deteriorations from a stable baseline
Aspirin-sensitive	May be associated with later onset and nasal polyps; 2–3% asthmatics on history but 10–20% on formal testing
Churg-Strauss syndrome	An uncommon diffuse vasculitis characterised by severe persistent asthma. The initial clue may be high eosinophilia (>1500/μl) or vasculitic involvement of another organ

tract infections. This pattern is often called 'intrinsic' asthma. Immediate skin prick tests are less likely to be positive because of a lack of involvement of allergens or a loss of skin test positivity with age.

Other categories

There are many patients who do not fit into these broad groups or who overlap the two types. Occupational asthma forms a subset where there is an identifiable cause which may work through an irritant or immunological trigger.

Some asthmatics are described as brittle, either with asthma that is uncontrolled with very variable obstruction (Type 1) or experiencing sudden deterioration from a background of good control (Type 2).

Presentation with cough is particularly common in children. Even in adults, asthma should be considered as the cause of chronic unexplained cough. In some series of such cases, asthma, or a combination of rhinitis and asthma, explained the cough in about half the patients who had been troubled by a cough with no obvious cause for more than 2 months.

Churg Strauss syndrome is a rare systemic vasculitis associated with asthma. The asthma is usually severe and often precedes other elements of the condition. The diagnostic criteria include asthma, blood and tissue eosinophilia and vasculitis. Treatment is with corticosteroids and other immunosuppressants, or any other treatment that is appropriate for the asthma which may be difficult to control.

References

Anderson HR, Gupta R, Strachan DP, Limb ES. 50 years of asthma: UK trends from 1955 to 2004. *Thorax* 2007; 62: 85–90.

Bateman ED, Hurd SS, Barnes PJ *et al.* Global strategy for asthma management and prevention. GINA executive summary. *European Respiratory Journal* 2008; 31: 143–178. http://www.ginasthma.com/Guidelineitem.asp??l1=2&l2=1&intId=1561.

Further reading

Anderson GP. Endotyping asthma: new insights into key pathogenic mechanisms in a complex heterogeneous disease. *Lancet* 2008; 372: 1107–1119.

CHAPTER 2

Prevalence

John Rees

Sherman Education Centre, Guy's Hospital, London, UK

OVERVIEW

- Genetic studies suggest that asthma is not a single disease but a collection of phenotypes with stronger genetic predisposition in earlier onset disease

- Prenatal stress, tobacco smoke and air pollutants have an effect on asthma risk

- The hygiene hypothesis links early exposure to infections from older siblings, animals and commensal gut bacteria to maturation of the immune system switching to a Th1 rather than Th2 lymphocyte phenotype

- For clinically significant asthma, many countries have broad prevalence rates of around 5% in adults and 10% in children

- Asthma increased for multiple reasons in developed countries but probably peaked in the early 1990s

Genetics

There have been considerable advances in understanding the genetics of asthma over the last few years. A familial link in asthma has been recognised for some time together with an association with allergic rhinitis and allergic eczema (Figure 2.1).

The familial link with atopic disorders is strongest in childhood asthma and with the link to maternal atopy. Earlier investigations were helped by the studies of isolated communities, such as Tristan da Cunha, where the high prevalence of asthma can be traced to three women among the original settlers.

Genetic studies

Early studies of genetic links within families with more than one subject with asthma showed promise of a strong link to certain genetic regions of interest. New genetic techniques have allowed genome-wide association studies. These have identified single nucleotide polymorphisms (SNPs) linked to asthma. More than 100 genes have now been implicated, each with a low attributable risk of less than 5%; the linkage does not mean that the genetic abnormality itself causes asthma. Various associations have been found such as SNPs in chromosome 17q21 linked to asthma developing under 4 years of age and associated with tobacco exposure(Bouzigon *et al.*, 2008). The SNPs span a number of genes. Susceptibility seems to be determined by a number of genes that have an effect on different aspects of asthma. These genetic studies suggest that asthma is not a single disease but a collection of phenotypes with stronger genetic predisposition in earlier onset disease.

It is unclear as to how the genetic variants identified cause asthma. Genes have been identified that are linked to the Th2 cytokine signalling pathway, Th2 cell differentiation, airway remodelling, innate and adaptive immune responses and immunoglobulin E (IgE) levels. Further research in this area may identify gene products that lead to new approaches to treatment and prevention.

Future investigations

Future investigations in the genetics of asthma may teach us more about susceptibility and progression in asthma. Genetic influences may also underlie different responses to treatment and raise the promise of matching treatment to a patient's individual response and the production of new forms of therapy aimed at influencing specific genes and their products.

Early environment

Genetic susceptibility alone does not account for the development or persistence of asthma (Figure 2.2). The genetic susceptibility

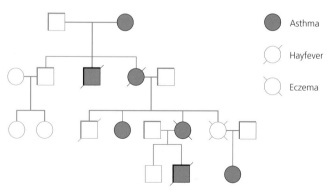

Asthma
Hayfever
Eczema

Figure 2.1 Family tree of an atopic family.

ABC of Asthma, 6th edition. By J. Rees, D. Kanabar and S. Pattani.
Published 2010 by Blackwell Publishing.

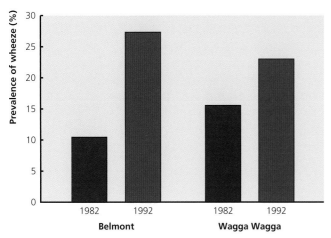

Figure 2.2 Increase in prevalence of wheeze in children aged 8–10 in two towns in New South Wales between 1982 and 1992. There was a pronounced increase in counts of house dust mite in domestic dust over the same period (Peat JK *et al.*, *British Medical Journal* 1994; 308: 1591–1596).

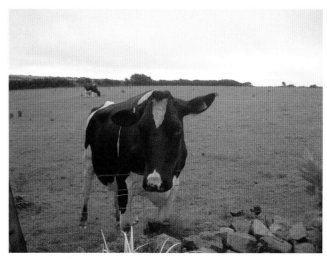

Figure 2.3 Early exposure to animals appears to reduce the risk of subsequent asthma.

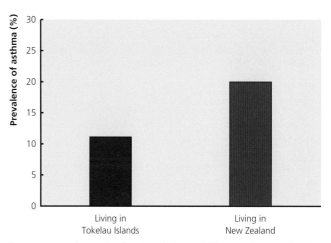

Figure 2.4 Prevalence of asthma in Tokelauan children aged 0–14 still in the Tokelau Islands or resettled to New Zealand. Asthma, rhinitis and eczema were all more prevalent in islanders who had settled in New Zealand after a hurricane. Environmental factors have an effect apart from genetic predisposition (Waite DA *et al.*, *Clinical Allergy* 1980; 10: 71–75).

is linked to environmental exposure. Even before birth, prenatal stress, tobacco smoke and air pollutants have an effect on asthma risk. Environmental influences before and soon after birth may be particularly important in the development of asthma. The type and extent of allergen exposure and infections may influence the development of the immune process and the likelihood of the development of asthma.

The *hygiene hypothesis* links to this balance of the parts of the immune system. It was noted that asthma was less likely to develop in children with older siblings. The hypothesis is that processes such as earlier exposure to infections from older siblings and commensal gut bacteria may help the maturation of the immune system and the switch to a Th1 lymphocyte phenotype rather than the Th2 phenotype. The Th1 cellular immune responses are related to protection against many infections, while Th2 responses favour atopy. This was supported by evidence that asthma and allergies are less common in children brought up on farms and in close contact with animals (Figure 2.3).

The hypothesis has been extended to suggest that, apart from immune maturation in infancy, the degree of competence of the immune system achieved at birth may be important. The influences on this are poorly understood but might be related to the prenatal cytokine environment.

Genetic factors and clinical course

Atopic subjects are at risk of asthma and rhinitis; they can be identified by positive immediate skin prick tests to common allergens.

The development of asthma depends on environmental factors acting with a genetic predisposition (Figure 2.4). The movement of racial groups with a low prevalence of asthma from an isolated rural environment to an urban area increases the prevalence in that group, possibly because of their increased exposure to allergens such as house dust mites and fungal spores or to infectious agents, pollution and dietary changes.

Family history

The chance of a person developing asthma by the age of 50 is increased 10 times if there is a first-degree relative with asthma. The risk is greater the more severe the relative's asthma is. It has been suggested that breastfeeding may reduce the risk of a child developing atopic conditions such as asthma because it restricts the exposure to ingested foreign protein in the first few months of life. Conflicting studies have been published and it may require considerable dietary restriction by the mother to avoid passing the antigen on to the child during this vulnerable period. Overall, although infant wheezing may be less common in breastfed infants, there is no good evidence to show that asthma is less prevalent in breastfed children. Nevertheless, many other benefits of breastfeeding indicate that it should be encouraged.

Smoking in pregnancy

Maternal smoking in pregnancy interferes with lung function development and increases the risk of childhood wheezing; exposure during the first few years of life is also detrimental. It is not clear that allergic conditions are increased. Studies of paternal smoking have shown less certain trends in the same direction.

Weight control

A number of studies have shown that obesity is associated with an increased likelihood of asthma, possibly through an effect of leptons on airway function. Regular exercise to maintain fitness and control weight is sensible advice for asthmatics.

Analgesics

Exposure to paracetamol emerged as a risk factor in some early epidemiological studies. This has been confirmed in the International Study of Asthma and Allergies in Childhood (ISAAC) study where paracetamol use in the first year of life does seem to be a risk factor for childhood asthma and for eczema and rhinoconjunctivitis (Beasley et al., 2008). The odds ratio was only 1.5 and explanations such as avoidance of aspirin and nonsteroidal anti-inflammatory drugs (NSAIDs) are possible alternatives.

Diagnostic criteria in epidemiological studies

For epidemiological purposes, a common set of criteria is the presence of symptoms during the previous 12 months, together with evidence of increased bronchial responsiveness. Phase 1 of ISAAC (Anderson et al., 2004) looked at prevalence of symptoms in 13- to 14-year-olds in 155 centres worldwide. Prevalence rates differed over 20-fold and ISAAC phase 2 explored these differences in more detail in 21 countries and suggested that atopy may be less important in less developed countries.

The Odense study (Siersted et al., 1996) in children found 27% with current asthma symptoms but only 10% were diagnosed as asthmatics. Different diagnostic tests such as methacholine responsiveness, peak flow monitoring and exercise testing did not correlate well with each other. Each test was reasonably specific but individual sensitivities tended to be low. In this study, the combination of peak flow monitoring at home and methacholine responsiveness produced the best results. The results confirm that no single physiological test is perfect and suggest that the different tests may detect different clinical aspects of asthma. A positive result in either test with a typical history would confirm the diagnosis of asthma.

Prevalence figures

The reported prevalence depends on the definition of asthma being used and the age and type of the population being studied. There are regional variations, particularly among developing countries where the rates in urban areas are higher than in the poor rural districts.

For clinically significant asthma, many countries have broad prevalence rates of around 5% in adults and 10% in children, but definitions based on hyper-responsiveness or wheeze in the last 12 months produce rates of around 30% in children.

In the past, it has been suggested that the label of asthma was used more readily in social classes I and II but more recent figures for young adults across Europe indicate a higher prevalence in lower socio-economic groups, regardless of their atopic status (Basagana et al., 2004).

Most studies using equivalent diagnostic criteria across the 1970s to 1990s showed that the prevalence of asthma was increasing. More recent studies show that this increase has reached a plateau or even reversed in developed countries (Figures 2.5 and 2.6). One recent study (Toelle et al., 2004) showed a decline from 29% to 24% in the symptom of wheeze over the past 12 months in Australian primary school children. The ISAAC showed a similar decrease from 34% to 28% for 12- to 14-year-olds between 1995 and 2002

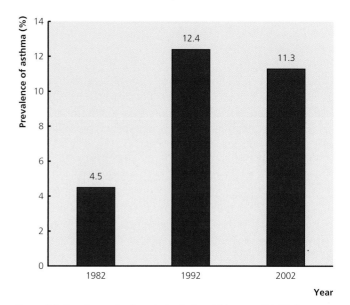

Figure 2.5 Prevalence of asthma in Australian children aged 8–11; the figure shows that the prevalence has reached a plateau (adapted with permission from Toelle BG, Ng K, Belousova E, Salome CM, Peat JK, Marks GB. Prevalence of asthma and allergy in schoolchildren in Belmont, Australia: three cross sectional surveys over 20 years. *British Medical Journal* 2004; 328: 386–387).

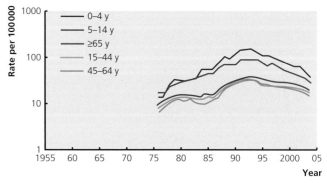

Figure 2.6 Mean weekly new episodes of asthma presenting to general practice, by age, England and Wales 1976–2004 (adapted from Anderson HR et al., *Thorax* 2007; 62: 85–90).

(Peat *et al.*, 1994). Interestingly, the label of asthma, especially mild asthma, was still increasing over this time.

During the last 10 years, admissions to hospital for asthma and emergency room attendances have declined, especially in children. This may be partly linked to better control through appropriate treatment. Overall, the pattern in developed countries suggests that prevalence peaked around 1990. Similar reductions have occurred in general practice (GP) consultations and in mortality of asthma. While there has been an increasing tendency to use the label of asthma, the true prevalence and the frequency of more serious asthma are showing signs of a reduction.

The sex ratio in children aged around 7 years shows that one and a half times to twice as many boys are affected as girls, but during their teenage years boys do better than girls and by the time they reach adulthood the sex incidence becomes almost equal.

Changes in prevalence

A number of explanations have been put forward for the increase in the prevalence of asthma. The strong genetic element has not changed, so any true increase outside changes in detection or diagnosis must come from environmental factors. No single explanation is likely to provide the complete answer since the likely factors do not apply equally to all the populations experiencing the change in prevalence. Explanations for the increase in the prevalence of asthma are discussed below.

Change in the indoor environment

The advent of centrally heated homes with warm bedrooms, high humidity and plentiful soft furnishings is likely to increase the exposure to house dust mite. This may be part of the explanation but does not fit with changes in developing countries.

Smoking

Maternal smoking during pregnancy and infancy is associated with an increased prevalence of asthma in childhood. The increase in smoking among young women in recent years may play some part in the increase in prevalence. Smoking by asthmatics increases the persistence of asthma.

Family size

First born children are more at risk of asthma and a general reduction in family size has increased the proportion of first born children.

Pollution

Symptoms of asthma are made worse by atmospheric pollutions such as nitrogen, sulphur dioxide and small particulate matter (Figure 2.7). However, outdoor environmental pollution levels do not correlate with changes in prevalence. Indoor pollution from oxides of nitrogen, organic compounds and fungal spores may play a more important role.

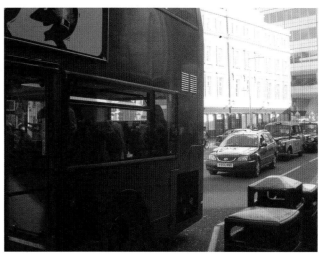

Figure 2.7 Outdoor pollution increases symptoms in existing asthmatics.

Diet

A number of studies have shown relationships between diet and asthma with respect to higher salt intake, low selenium or reduced vitamin C, vitamin E or certain polysaturated fats. However, the effects of dietary intervention do not support this as a major contribution. In conclusion, the prevalence changes in the latter part of the twentieth century were widespread and genuine. No single factor explains changes or the end of the rise in recent years.

References

Anderson HR, Ruggles R, Strachan DP *et al.* Trends in prevalence of symptoms of asthma, hay fever, and eczema in 12–14 year olds in the British Isles, 1995–2002: questionnaire survey. *British Medical Journal* 2004; 328: 1052–1053.

Basagana X, Sunyer J, Kogevinas M *et al.* Socio-economic status and asthma prevalence in young adults: the European community health survey. *American Journal of Epidemiology* 2004; 160: 178–188.

Beasley R, Clayton T, Crane J *et al.* Association between paracetamol use in infancy and childhood and risk of asthma, rhinoconjunctivitis, and eczema in children aged 6–7 years: analysis from Phase Three of the ISAAC programme. *Lancet* 2008; 372: 1039–1048.

Bouzigon E, Corda E, Aschard H *et al.* Effect of 17q21 variants and smoking exposure on early-onset asthma. *The New England Journal of Medicine* 2008; 359: 1985–1994.

Peat JK, van den Berg RH, Green WF, Mellis CM, Leeder SR, Woolcock AJ. Changing prevalence of asthma in Australian children. *British Medical Journal* 1994; 308: 1591–1596.

Siersted HC, Mostgaard G, Hyldebrandt N, Hansen HS, Boldsen J, Oxho JH. Interrelationships between diagnosed asthma, asthma-like symptoms, and abnormal airway behaviour in adolescence: the Odense School child Study. *Thorax* 1996; 51: 503–509.

Toelle BG, Ng K, Belousova E, Salome CM, Peat JK, Marks GB. Prevalence of asthma and allergy in schoolchildren in Belmont, Australia: three cross sectional surveys over 20 years. *British Medical Journal* 2004; 328: 386–387.

Further reading

Anderson HR, Gupta R, Strachan DP, Limb ES. 50 years of asthma: UK trends from 1955 to 2004. *Thorax* 2007; 62: 85–90.

CHAPTER 3

Diagnostic Testing and Monitoring

John Rees

Sherman Education Centre, Guy's Hospital, London, UK

OVERVIEW

- Mini peak flow meters provide a simple method of measuring airflow obstruction
- Every patient should have a written personal asthma management plan
- The typical variability of asthma can be assessed by peak flow variation with time or bronchodilator, or by provocation by exercise, histamine or methacholine
- Specific allergic triggers are assessed through a combination of careful history and skin test or measurement of specific immunoglobulin E (IgE)
- 'All that wheezes is not asthma' – alternative diagnoses should be considered in atypical cases
- Standard questions such as the Royal College of Physicians' three questions or the asthma control test are useful in monitoring control

Recording airflow obstruction

Mini peak flow meters provide a simple method of measuring airflow obstruction.

The measurements add an objective element to subjective feelings of shortness of breath. Several types of meters are available. The traditional Wright peak flow meters had errors that varied over the range of measurement (Figure 3.1). Since patients use the same peak flow meter over time, they can build up a pattern of their asthma, which can be important in changing their treatment and planning management. From September 2004, meters became available with a new scale giving accurate readings over the full range. They compare accurately with peak flow values from other sources such as spirometry. Some patients may still have meters with the old scale.

Use of diary cards

Although acute attacks of asthma occasionally have a sudden catastrophic onset, they are more usually preceded by a gradual deterioration in control, which may not be noticed until it is

ABC of Asthma, 6th edition. By J. Rees, D. Kanabar and S. Pattani.
Published 2010 by Blackwell Publishing.

quite advanced. A few patients, probably 15–20%, are unaware of moderate changes in their airflow obstruction even when these occur acutely; these patients are at particular risk of an acute exacerbation without warning (Box 3.1). When such patients are identified, they should be encouraged to take regular peak flow recordings and enter them on a diary card, to permit them to see trends in peak flow measurements and react to exacerbations at an early stage before there is any change in their symptoms.

> Box 3.1 **Priorities in peak flow recording**
>
> Particular encouragement to record peak flow should be given to the following patients:
>
> - Poor perceivers, where symptoms do not reflect changes in objective measured obstruction
> - Patients with a history of sudden exacerbations
> - Patients with poor asthma control
> - Times of adjustment in therapy either up or down
> - Situations where a link to a precipitating factor is suspected
> - Periodic recordings in stable asthma to establish usual levels and confirm reliability of symptoms

Written asthma action plans

Mini peak flow meters are inexpensive and have an important role in educating patients about their asthma. Simply giving out a peak flow meter, however, has little benefit. Using home recordings, the doctor or nurse and patient can work together to develop plans with criteria that indicate the need for a change in treatment, a visit to the doctor or emergency admission to hospital. This management plan should be agreed upon and written down for the patient and should then be reviewed periodically. It should be based on the patient's best peak flow value. Peak flow can help the patient to interpret the severity of symptoms and need for help.

It has not been possible to show an effect on the control of asthma or hospital admission from the use of a peak flow meter alone, but a written personal asthma management plan supported by regular follow-up does improve control. These have been shown to help reduce emergency attendances, hospital admissions and lung function. They should show the patient what to do, when to do it, for how long, and when further medical advice is needed.

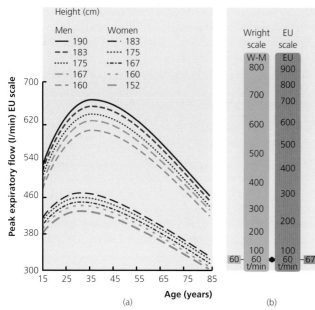

Height (cm)

Men	Women
—— 190	— · 183
– – 183	· · · · · 175
· · · · · 175	– · – 167
– – 167	– – 160
– – 160	— 152

Figure 3.1 (a) Normal range of peak flow varies with gender, age and height. (b) Mini Wright new scale. Errors in readings of Mini-Wright and Wright peak flow meters compared with flow from a pneumotachograph. Both over-read at lower flow rates and are non-linear (Miller *et al.*, 1992). Peak flow meters meeting the new European standard EN13826 with an accurate peak flow measurement have been available since September 2004. Miller MR, Dickinson SA, Hitchings DJ *Thorax* 1992; 47: 904–909.

Responsiveness to bronchodilators

Responses to bronchodilators are easy to measure in the clinic or surgery: Reversibility can be useful in establishing the diagnosis of asthma where there is doubt (Figure 3.2). Because of the variability in asthma, airflow obstruction may not be present at the time of testing. Reversibility is relatively specific but not very sensitive as a diagnostic test in mild asthma. Testing to find out the most effective bronchodilator is less helpful since acute responses are not necessarily predictive of long-term effects.

Measuring reversibility

Reversibility is usually assessed by recording the best of three peak flow measurements and repeating the   measurements

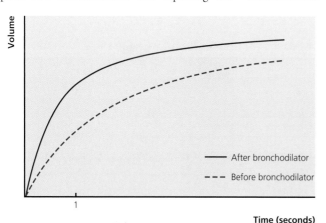

Figure 3.2 Reversibility in asthma shown by change in FEV_1 on spirometry.

15–30 minutes after the patient has inhaled two or more doses of a β-agonist, salbutamol or terbutaline, from a metered dose inhaler or dry powder system. The method of inhalation should be supervised and the opportunity taken to correct the technique or change to a different inhalation device, if necessary. The 95% confidence intervals for a change in peak flow rate on such repetitions are around 60 1/minute, and it is usual to look for a change in peak flow of 20% and 60 1/minute.

When forced expiratory volume in one second (FEV_1) is the measurement used, a change of 200 ml is outside the variability of the test. Changes of this size are not unusual in chronic obstructive pulmonary disease (COPD) but a change of >400 ml in FEV_1 is highly suggestive of asthma. A standard dose of a β-agonist can be combined with an anticholinergic agent – ipratropium bromide. These agents are slower to act than β-agonists and their effect should be assessed 40–60 minutes after inhalation.

When there is severe obstruction and reversibility is limited, application of strict reversibility criteria may be correct for diagnosis but inappropriate for the purpose of determining treatments since 20% of a very low peak flow or FEV_1 is within the error of the test. Any response may be worthwhile; therefore attention should be paid to subjective responses and improvement of exercise tolerance, together with results of other tests of respiratory function. Reversibility shown by other tests, such as those of lung volumes or trapped gas volumes without changes in peak flow or FEV_1, are more likely to occur in patients with COPD than in those with asthma.

When making changes in treatment, such as the introduction of long-acting β-agonists, it is important to evaluate the effects of these interventions. Peak expiratory flow recording is an important evaluation tool usually combined with other measures such as symptoms or use of short-acting reliever bronchodilators.

Further review

Decisions about treatment from such single-dose studies should be backed up by further objective and subjective measurements during long-term treatment. Responses to bronchodilators are not necessarily consistent and, in some patients, changes after single doses in the laboratory may not predict the responses to the same drug over prolonged periods.

Peak flow variation

Characteristic of asthma is a cyclical variation in the degree of airflow obstruction throughout the day (Figure 3.3). The lowest peak flow values occur in the early hours of the morning and the highest occur in the afternoon. To see the pattern, a peak flow meter should be used at least twice and up to four times a day, taking the best of three measurements on each occasion. Possible reasons for the variation include diurnal variation in adrenaline, vagal activity, cortisol, airway inflammation and changes in $β_2$-receptor function. Variation may also be caused by occupational or other environmental exposure or poor adherence to therapy.

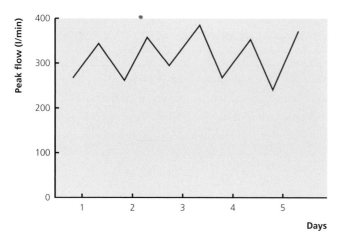

Figure 3.3 Diurnal percentage variation in peak flow readings. Amplitude best is >20% each day.

Diurnal variation

Documentation of diurnal variation by recording measurements from a peak flow meter shows typical diagnostic patterns in many patients. The timing of the measurements should be recorded; otherwise typical variations can be obscured by later readings at the weekend or on days away from work or school. Variation has been calculated in a number of different ways. Percentage amplitude best is calculated as (highest − lowest)/highest × 100. Amplitude best of 20% on 3 days of two consecutive weeks is likely to mean that asthma is present but changes smaller than this do not exclude asthma and the sensitivity is only around 25%. In people without asthma, there is a small degree of diurnal variation with the same timing.

Nocturnal attacks

People with asthma commonly complain of waking up at night (Figure 3.4). Large studies in the United Kingdom suggest that more than half of those with asthma have their sleep disturbed by an

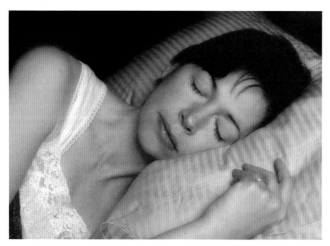

Figure 3.4 The lowest peak flow values occur in the early hours of the morning.

attack more than once a week. Questions about sleep disturbance by breathlessness and cough should be asked routinely in consultations with asthmatic patients. Deaths from asthma are also more likely to occur in the early hours of the morning.

Exercise testing

The provocation test most often used in the United Kingdom is a simple exercise test (Box 3.2). Exercise testing is a safe, simple procedure and may be useful when the diagnosis of asthma is in doubt (Figure 3.5). Non-asthmatic patients do not develop bronchoconstriction on exercise; indeed, they usually show a small degree of bronchodilatation during the exercise itself. When baseline lung function is low, provocation testing is unnecessary for diagnosis as reversibility can be shown by bronchodilatation.

> Box 3.2 **Exercise test**
>
> An exercise test may consist of baseline peak flow measurements, then 6 minutes of vigorous supervised exercise such as running, followed by peak flow measurements for 30 minutes afterwards.

Exercise testing and the recording of diurnal variations are used when the history suggests asthma but lung function is normal when the patient is seen. It is less sensitive but more easily available than histamine or methacholine challenge test.

Testing outdoors

The exercise is best done outside because breathing cold, dry air intensifies the response. The characteristic asthmatic response is a fall in peak flow of more than 15% several minutes after the end of 6–8 minute exercise. About 90% of asthmatic children will show a drop in peak flow in response to exercise but responses are reduced by treatment. Once the peak flow rate has fallen by 15%, the bronchoconstriction should be reversed by inhalation of a bronchodilator. Occurrence of late reactions hours after the challenge is unusual unlike in the case of challenge with an allergen. Patients do not need to be kept under observation for late responses

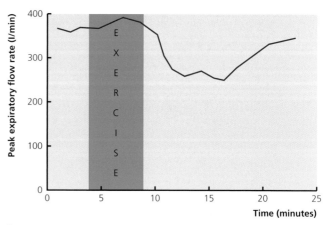

Figure 3.5 Decrease in peak expiratory flow rate in response to exercise.

after the initial response has been reversed. Such tests are best avoided if the patient has ischaemic heart disease, but there is no reason why peak flow measurements should not be included during supervised exercise testing for coronary artery disease where this is appropriate.

Bronchodilators and sodium cromoglicate should be stopped at least 6 hours before the exercise test and long-acting oral or inhaled bronchodilators and β-antagonists should be stopped for at least 24 hours. Prolonged use of inhaled corticosteroids reduces responses to exercise but these are not stopped before testing because the effect takes days or weeks to wear off.

Other types of challenge

The exercise test relies on changes in temperature and in the osmolality of the airway mucosa. Other challenge tests that rely on similar mechanisms include isocapnic hyperventilation; breathing cold, dry air; and osmotic challenge with nebulised distilled water or hypertonic saline. These are, however, laboratory-based procedures rarely used in practice.

Airway hyper-responsiveness

Other common forms of non-specific challenge to the airways are the inhalation of methacholine and histamine. These tests produce a range of responses usually defined as the dose of the challenging agent necessary to produce a drop in the FEV_1 of 20%. This is calculated by giving increasing doses until the FEV_1 drops below 80% of the baseline measurement, then drawing a line to connect the last two points above and below a 20% drop and taking the dose at the point on this line equivalent to a 20% drop in FEV_1 (Figure 3.6). Nearly all patients with asthma show increased responsiveness, whereas patients with hay fever, and not asthma, form an intermediate group.

This responsiveness of asthmatic patients has been associated with the underlying inflammation in the airway wall. Such non-specific bronchial challenge is performed as an outpatient procedure in hospital respiratory function units. It is a safe procedure, provided it is monitored carefully and not used in the presence of moderately severe airflow obstruction.

Hyper-responsiveness may occur in conditions such as rhinitis, bronchiectasis and COPD. It would be unusual, however, to sustain the diagnosis of asthma in a patient with normal airway responsiveness on no treatment.

Degree of responsiveness

The degree of responsiveness is associated with the severity of the airway disease. It can be reduced by strict avoidance of known allergens. Drugs such as corticosteroids reduce responsiveness through their effect on inflammation in the wall of the airway but they do not usually return reactivity to the normal range. Use of a bronchodilator is followed by a temporary reduction while the mechanisms of smooth muscle contraction are blocked. Bronchial reactivity is an important epidemiological and research tool. In clinical practice, its use varies widely between countries. It is most useful where there are difficult diagnostic problems such as persistent cough.

Specific airway challenge

Challenge with specific agents to which a patient is thought to be sensitive must be done with caution. The initial dose should be low and, even so, reactions may be unpredictable. Early narrowing of the airway by contraction of smooth muscle occurs within the first 30 minutes and there is often a 'late response' after 4–8 hours (Figure 3.7).

The late response may be followed by poorer control of the asthma and greater diurnal variation for days or weeks afterwards. The late response is thought to be associated with release of mediators and attraction of inflammatory cells to the airways. It has been used in drug development as a more suitable model for clinical asthma than the brief early response.

Challenges with specific allergens are used mostly for the investigation of occupational asthma but they should be restricted to experienced laboratories. Patients should be supervised for at least 8 hours after challenge.

Skin tests

In skin prick tests, a small amount of the test substance is introduced into the superficial layers of the epidermis through the tip of a small

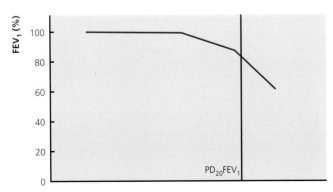

Figure 3.6 Log dose of histamine or methacholine.

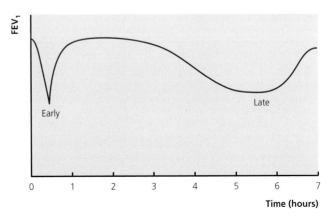

Figure 3.7 Drop in FEV_1 in a bronchial reactivity test.

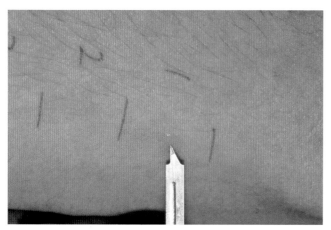

Figure 3.8 Skin prick tests. This patient is being tested for responses to a range of common allergens.

needle (Figure 3.8). The tests are painless, just causing temporary local itching. More generalised reactions are theoretically possible but extremely rare. Most young asthmatics show a range of positive responses to common environmental allergens such as house dust mite, pollens and animal dander. A weal 3 mm larger than the negative control that develops 15 minutes after a skin prick test suggests the presence of specific immunoglobulin E (IgE) antibody; the results correlate well with those of *in vitro* tests for IgE such as the radioallergosorbent test (RAST) which is more expensive but may be helpful in difficult cases in the presence of widespread asthma.

Atopy

Positive skin tests do not establish a diagnosis of asthma or the importance of the specific allergens used. They show only the tendency to produce IgE to common allergens confirming atopy. More than 20% of the population have positive skin tests, but less than half of these will develop asthma. The prevalence and strength of positive skin tests decline with age. The pattern of skin test responses depends on prior exposure and, therefore, varies with geography and social factors.

Importance of history

The importance of allergic factors in asthma is best ascertained from a careful clinical history, taking into account seasonal factors and trials of avoidance of allergens. Suspicions can be confirmed by skin tests, RAST or, less often, by specific inhalation challenge.

Conclusions

Although positive skin tests do not incriminate the allergen as a cause of the patient's asthma, it would be rare for an inhalant to be important in asthma with a negative result. The results do, however, rely on the quality of the agents used in testing and will be negative if antihistamines or leukotriene receptor antagonists are being taken. Bronchodilators and corticosteroids have no appreciable effect on immediate skin prick tests.

Differential diagnosis in adults

The difficulty in breathing that is characteristic of asthma may be described as a constriction in the chest that suggests ischaemic cardiac pain. Nocturnal asthma that causes the patient to be woken from sleep because of breathlessness may be confused with the paroxysmal nocturnal dyspnoea of heart failure.

Asthma and COPD

After some years, particularly when it is severe, asthma may lose some or all of its reversibility. COPD, usually caused by cigarette smoking, may show appreciable reversibility, which can make it quite difficult to be sure of the correct diagnosis in older patients with partially reversible obstruction. The pathological changes in the airway are different in asthma and COPD.

However, in practice, bronchodilators are given and corticosteroids are often used to establish the best airway function that can be achieved. Inhaled corticosteroids are more important in asthma treatment than in COPD. When there is reversibility to bronchodilators and any doubt whether the diagnosis might be asthma, inhaled corticosteroids should be part of the treatment.

Non-asthmatic wheezing

Other causes of wheezing, such as obstruction of the large airways, occasionally produce problems in diagnosis. This may be the case with foreign bodies, particularly in children, or with tumours that gradually obstruct the trachea or main airways in adults. The noise produced is often a single-pitched wheeze on inspiration and expiration rather than the multiple expiratory wheezes typical of widespread narrowing in asthma.

Appropriate X-rays and flow volume loops can show the site of obstruction. On a flow volume curve a fixed low flow will be evident (Figure 3.9), while on spirometry the volume–time curve may be a straight line.

Vocal cord dysfunction

Some patients have upper airway obstruction at laryngeal level produced apparently by dysfunction of the vocal cord musculature.

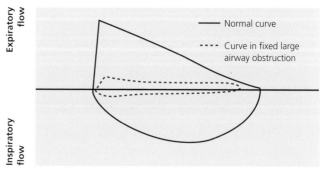

Figure 3.9 Flow volume loop in fixed large airway obstruction.

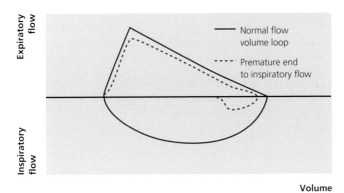

Figure 3.10 Flow volume loop in vocal cord dysfunction.

The obstruction is most evident in inspiration and may show as premature termination of inspiration in the flow volume loop (Figure 3.10). The phenomenon seems to be more common in young women; it is often mistaken for, or coincident with, asthma and can be difficult to treat.

Hyperventilation syndrome

The sensation of dyspnoea and an inability to take a full inspiration are characteristic of hyperventilation and may be confused with asthma. The diagnosis relies on a careful history and can be confirmed by measurement of breathing pattern, carbon dioxide in arterial blood or exhaled air at rest or on response to voluntary hyperventilation. Acute asthma attacks are frightening and hyperventilation may occur with asthma or be confused with the same. Always err on the side of caution in treating such patients.

Monitoring asthma control

Peak expiratory flow

As described earlier, this is particularly useful in detecting triggers, such as occupation, assessing treatment response and in helping the patient confirm change in symptoms.

Symptoms

It is important to evaluate symptoms with specific questions on breathlessness, cough and night-time wakening. This can be done systematically with the Royal College of Physicians' three questions (Table 3.1), the asthma control questionnaire (see Further reading) or the asthma control test (Table 3.2). These allow a quantitative assessment useful for comparison and for audit. Symptoms may be recorded on diary cards.

Exacerbations

Exacerbations should be regarded as a failure of control and prompt an evaluation of the circumstances, the patient's treatment, compliance and response to the start of any deterioration.

Table 3.1 The Royal College of Physicians' three questions on asthma control.

In the last week/month		
Have you had difficulty sleeping because of asthma symptoms (including cough)?	Yes	No
Have you had your usual asthma symptoms during the day (cough, wheeze, chest tightness or breathlessness)?	Yes	No
Has your asthma interfered with your normal activities (e.g. housework, work, school etc)?	Yes	No

Table 3.2 Asthma control test.

In the past *4 weeks*, how much of the time did your *asthma* keep you from getting as much done at work, school or at home?				
All of the time	Most of the time	Some of the time	A little of the time	None of the time
1	2	3	4	5
During the past *4 weeks*, how often have you had shortness of breath?				
More than once a day	Once a day	3–6 times a week	Once or twice a week	Not at all
1	2	3	4	5
During the past *4 weeks*, how often did your *asthma* symptoms (wheezing, coughing, shortness of breath, chest tightness or pain) wake you up at night or earlier than usual in the morning?				
Four or more nights a week	Two or three times a week	Once a week	Once or twice	Not at all
1	2	3	4	5
During the past *4 weeks*, how often have you used your rescue inhaler or nebuliser medication (such as salbutamol)?				
Three or more times a day	One or two times a day	Two or three times a week	Once or twice a week	Not at all
1	2	3	4	5
How would you rate your *asthma* control during the *past 4 weeks*?				
Not controlled at all	Poorly controlled	Somewhat controlled	Well controlled	Completely controlled
1	2	3	4	5

If you scored 19 or less, it may be an indication that your asthma is not under control. Make an appointment to discuss your Asthma Control Test score with your doctor and ask if you should change your asthma treatment plan.

Bronchodilator use

Use of short-acting bronchodilators reflects asthma control and the patient's response. This can be assessed from the patient's account, diary cards or prescribing data.

Expired air

Measurement of exhaled NO has become a practical measurement linked to airway inflammation. It reflects response to steroid therapy but values vary widely and it has not yet found a practical role in routine monitoring.

Eosinophils

Measurement of sputum eosinophilia has been shown to help in controlling asthma while limiting inhaled corticosteroid use and reducing exacerbations. However, it is not practical for the great majority of asthmatics but could be replaced by a simpler, portable measure of expired air.

Further reading

Jones K, Cleary R, Hyland M. Predictive value of a simple asthma morbidity index in a general practice population. *British Journal of General Practice* 1999; 49: 23–26.

Juniper EF, Guyatt GH, Cox FM, Ferrie PJ, King DR. Development and validation of the Mini Asthma Quality of Life Questionnaire. *European Respiratory Journal* 1999; 14: 32–38.

Szefler SJ, Mitchell H, Sorkness CA *et al*. Management of asthma based on exhaled nitric oxide in addition to guideline-based treatment for inner-city adolescents and young adults: a randomised controlled trial. *Lancet* 2008; 372: 1065–1072.

Toelle BG, Ram FS. Written individualised management plans for asthma in children and adults. *Cochrane Database of Systematic Reviews* 2004; (2): CD002171.

Asthma UK's free 'be in control' pack contains an asthma review card, a peak flow diary, a personal asthma action plan and a medicine card and is available at http://www.asthma.org.uk/all_about_asthma/publications/index.html

CHAPTER 4

Clinical Course

John Rees

Sherman Education Centre, Guy's Hospital, London, UK

OVERVIEW

- Over half the children whose wheezing is infrequent will be free of symptoms by the time they are 21 years old
- Only 20% of children with frequent, troublesome wheezing will be symptom free at 21
- Boys are more likely to have asthma than girls but more likely to grow out of it
- Mortality due to asthma is related to inadequate treatment, poor response to deterioration and adverse psychosocial factors
- Educating patients about their asthma and the use of treatment is an integral part of management

'Growing out' of asthma

Parents of asthmatic children are usually concerned about whether their child will 'grow out' of asthma. Most wheezy children improve during their teens but the outlook depends to some extent on the severity of their early disease.

Over half the children whose wheezing is infrequent will be free of symptoms by the time they are 21 years old, but of those with frequent, troublesome wheezing only 20% will be symptom free at 21, although 20% will be substantially better. In 15% of patients, asthma becomes more troublesome in early adult years than it was in childhood. Even if there is prolonged remission lasting several years, symptoms may return later (Sears *et al.*, 2003). In a New Zealand study, wheezing was persistent in 14.5% of children up to age 26, while 12.4% wheezed in childhood, remitted and then relapsed by age 26 (Stern *et al.*, 2008). After months free of symptoms, biopsy studies show that the airway epithelium may still be inflamed and airway responsiveness to methacholine and histamine may remain abnormally high. This suggests that the underlying tendency to be asthmatic remains.

ABC of Asthma, 6th edition. By J. Rees, D. Kanabar and S. Pattani.
Published 2010 by Blackwell Publishing.

Likelihood of remission

Asthma is less likely to go into remission in patients with a strong family history of atopy or a personal history of other atopic conditions, low respiratory function, onset after the age of 29 and frequent attacks. More boys than girls are affected by asthma, but the girls do less well during adolescence, and by adulthood the sex ratio is equal. Most of those who do grow out of asthma are left with no residual effects other than the risk of recrudescence. Smoking increases the likelihood of persistence, while an early onset is predictive of relapse. Other predictors of adult asthma are Alternaria and house dust mite sensitivity, hyper-responsiveness and low lung function.

In those with persistent asthma through childhood respiratory function tests are significantly reduced. Chest deformities are uncommon and only occur when there is severe, intractable disease.

Adult height

Although puberty may be delayed, the final adult height of children with asthma is usually normal unless they have received long-term treatment with systemic or high-dose inhaled corticosteroids.

Prognosis in adults

New diagnoses of asthma in adults are more common in women. Asthma in adults often shows less spontaneous variation than it does in children. Wheezing is more persistent and there is less association with obvious precipitating factors other than infections. The chances of a sustained remission are also lower than in children. Smokers with increased bronchial reactivity are particularly at risk of developing chronic airflow obstruction and it is vital that asthmatic patients do not smoke. When there are known precipitating agents that can be avoided – such as animals or occupational factors – then sustained removal of these can reduce bronchial reactivity. The avoidance of contact with known allergens can decrease the inflammation in the airway wall and thus reduce responses to non-specific agents including cigarette smoke, cold air and dust. It can lead to an improvement in the control and the progress of the asthma (Box 4.1).

Box 4.1 **Definition of control of asthma**

No day-time symptoms
No night-time wakening due to asthma
No need for rescue medication
No exacerbations
No limitation of activity including exercise
Normal lung function
Minimal side effects

(From British Guideline on the Management of Asthma. Thorax 2008; 63 (Supplement IV).)

The reversibility of airway obstruction in asthma is not always maintained throughout life. Those with more severe asthma are most likely to go on to develop irreversible airflow obstruction. It is likely that this progression to irreversibility is related to persistent inflammation of the wall of the airway, which leads to permanent damage through remodelling of the airway wall. Suitable prolonged prophylaxis reduces the inflammation and most chest physicians act on the belief that this will reduce the likelihood of long-term damage and eventual irreversibility. There are few prolonged studies to prove or disprove this contention, but the benefits of anti-inflammatory prophylaxis are well-established in the short term and it seems prudent to follow this practice.

A few studies on introduction of inhaled corticosteroids give some hope that treatment can affect the clinical course. The degree of impairment in lung function on starting inhaled steroids is greatest in those with the longest history of symptoms, suggesting that more prolonged untreated disease may lead to irreversible change (Figure 4.1). Delayed onset of inhaled steroids in one study comparing β-agonists and steroids seemed to reduce the potential benefit of the steroids. Set against these studies are the changes seen at the end of trials of inhaled steroids. Bronchial responsiveness and lung function seem to return to baseline rapidly on stopping treatment.

Important areas for further study with implications for the stage to start inhaled steroids include the relative position of bronchodilators, steroids and other agents such as cromoglycate, theophylline and leukotriene antagonists in treatment, the degree of control that is looked for and the approach to treatment once control is achieved.

Severe exacerbations may lead to decline in lung function and this may be attenuated by the use of inhaled steroids reducing exacerbations.

Deaths from asthma

Since the sharp temporary increase in mortality from asthma seen in some countries during the early 1960s, there has been concern about the role of treatment in such deaths. The deaths in the 1960s have been attributed to cardiac stimulation caused by overuse of inhaled isoprenaline or to excessive reliance on its usual efficacy leading to delay in using appropriate alternative treatment when symptoms worsened. Isoprenaline as a bronchodilator has been superseded by safer β2-stimulants, although excess deaths in New Zealand in the 1990s may have had a similar cause.

After the peak in the 1960s, the number of deaths from asthma in the United Kingdom stabilised (Figure 4.2). In the late 1980s, there was a suggestion of a gradual rise in deaths to about 2000 per year but statistics for the 1990s show a gradual decline in mortality (Figure 4.2). The figures are most reliable for the 5- to 34-year age range and the most recent figures confirm a slight fall in mortality in the group. Confidential enquiries into deaths suggest that clinical management issues have reduced while patient factors such as compliance and psychosocial problems have become more important (Campbell *et al.*, 1997).

A few deaths occur after inappropriate use of β-blockers or a nonsteroidal anti-inflammatory drug in sensitive patients.

Need for rapid response

Investigation of the circumstances surrounding individual deaths generally finds evidence of under-treatment rather than excessive

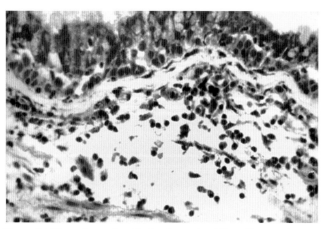

Figure 4.1 Biopsy from asthmatic showing eosinophilia and increased thickness of basement membrane (courtesy of Professor Chris Corrigan).

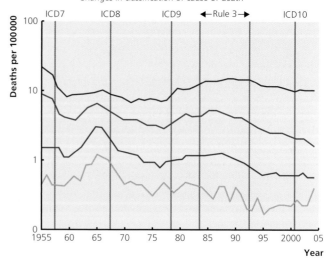

Figure 4.2 Deaths from asthma in England and Wales by age group (adapted from Anderson HR, Gupta R, Strachan DP, Limb ES. 50 years of asthma: UK trends from 1955 to 2004. *Thorax* 2007; 62: 85–90).

medication in such deaths. Most deaths occur in patients with chronic severe asthma. Doctors and patients underestimate the severity of attacks; the most important factor may be an apparent reluctance to take oral corticosteroids for severe asthmatic episodes and to adjust treatment early during periods of deterioration. Nevertheless, a minority of deaths occur less than an hour after the start of an exacerbation. Patients who have such rapid deterioration are particularly vulnerable. If patients have deteriorated swiftly in the past they should have suitable treatment readily available, such as steroids and nebulised and injectable bronchodilators. Patients and their relatives must be confident in the use of their emergency treatment and know how to obtain further help immediately.

Several centres have adopted the policy of maintaining a self-admission service for selected asthmatic patients. This avoids delay in admitting patients to hospital and is a logical development towards involving patients in the management of their own disease.

Diurnal variation

Some studies have shown that patients are particularly at risk after they have been discharged from intensive care or high dependency units to ordinary wards, and after discharge from hospital. Problems often occur in the early hours of the morning at the nadir of the diurnal cycle. They may be related to premature tailing off of the initial intensive treatment because the measurements during the day have been satisfactory. Monitoring of peak flow will identify the instability of the asthma manifested by a large diurnal variability in peak flow. Adequate supervision and treatment must be maintained throughout these periods until control is restored.

Inpatient management

Assessment and management in hospital have also been criticised. Asthma has proved to be a popular subject for audit according to the consensus guidelines of the British Thoracic Society (BTS), and the Scottish Intercollegiate Guidelines Network (SIGN) studies have shown that initial assessment and treatment are satisfactory but that there are weaknesses in the exploration of reasons for an attack, establishment of adequate control before discharge and follow-up arrangements. Meeting the criteria of peak expiratory flow (PEF) >75% best or predicated and diurnal variability <25% and establishment of a personalised management plan are the commonest problems in audits of asthma care. Every admission should be regarded as a failure of routine management. The usual treatment, compliance with therapy and the existence and performance of management plans should be explored with the patient. Quality of treatment, readmission rates and asthma control are improved when the inpatient care is supervised by those with an interest in thoracic medicine. Admission to hospital is an appropriate opportunity to involve a respiratory nurse specialist in the management.

Morbidity

Asthma causes considerable morbidity with persistent symptoms and loss of time from work and school. Repeated studies have shown that the aims of most guidelines are not met in a large proportion of patients. In milder disease (steps 1–3 of the BTS guidelines) the aim is perfect control although patient preferences need to be taken into account. Such control is achieved in less than half the patients in practice, which suggests that the expectations of many doctors and patients are not high enough. Sleep is disturbed by asthma more than once a week in over 50% of patients and this leads to poorer day-time performance. There has been a shift in the general approach to management aiming to produce freedom from symptoms, rather than a tolerable existence free of disabling attacks. The aims of the first three steps of the BTS guidelines involve virtual freedom from symptoms with minimal or no use of rescue bronchodilator. In children, this would include freedom to take part in regular exercise. This requires a more aggressive approach early in the course of the disease with regular anti-inflammatory drugs and will, it is hoped, lead to a reduction in morbidity from exacerbations of asthma and long-term damage.

Asthma is classified in different ways depending on the level of control and treatment. In the British Guidelines, classification is based on the level of the treatment step that is needed to maintain control. In the GINA guidelines, it is based on the prevalence of symptoms and lung function before treatment starts and then control is defined in three levels (see Table 4.1 and Box 4.1). In general, it is more helpful to think of severity in terms of the level of treatment needed to establish good control. Control is the level of symptoms occurring on treatment combined with the risk of future problems such as exacerbations and irreversible obstruction.

Patient education

Educating patients about their asthma and the use of treatment is an integral part of management. Internet sources from the Lung and Asthma Information Agency (www.laia.ac.uk) and Asthma UK (www.asthma.org.uk) provide useful reliable information (Box 4.2). Patients forget much of what they are told in consultations and hence information should be backed up by written instructions.

Table 4.1 Classification of asthma.

Characteristic	Controlled (All of the following)	Partly controlled (Any measure present in any week)	Uncontrolled
Day-time symptoms	None (twice or less/week)	More than twice/week	Three or more features of partly controlled asthma present in any week
Limitations of activities	None	Any	
Nocturnal symptoms/ awakening	None	Any	
Need for reliever/rescue treatment	None (twice or less/week)	More than twice/week	
Lung function (PEF or FEV$_1$)	Normal	80% predicted or personal best (if known)	
Exacerbations	None	One or more/year	One in any week

FEV$_1$, forced expiratory volume in 1 second.
(From Bateman ED, Hurd SS, Barnes PJ *et al.* Global strategy for asthma management and prevention: GINA executive summary. *The European Respiratory Journal* 2008; 31: 143–178).

It is often helpful to produce these individually for each patient. Standard written information from asthma societies and other sources can be used as a backup, but a personal plan is preferable and can be produced from simple word processor templates. Patients are often confused about basic aspects such as the differences between regular prophylaxis with inhaled corticosteroids or sodium cromoglycate, and the quickly effective inhaled bronchodilators used to treat acute attacks.

Box 4.2 **Asthma UK**

Asthma UK is a charity dedicated to improving the health and well-being of people in the United Kingdom, whose lives are affected by asthma.

> Website: www.asthma.org.uk
> Advice line: 08457 01 02 03
> People can email an asthma nurse specialist at www.asthma.org.uk/adviceline

---

Availability of a mini peak flow meter and standardised definitions of control allow the patient to participate more effectively in the understanding and treatment of the disease. Even with this information, though, many patients do not adhere to their prescribed regimen. Only half of all asthmatic patients achieve 75% compliance with their prescribed treatment. This is true for all chronic conditions and shows the need for regular reinforcement (matching the information to the patients) and for further work in the area of education and compliance. Development of these management plans requires time, reinforcing and extending the information on repeat visits.

References

Campbell MJ, Cogman GR, Holgate ST, Johnston SL. Age specific trends in asthma mortality in England and Wales, 1983–1995: results of an observational study. *British Medical Journal* 1997; 314: 1439–1441.

Sears MR, Greene JM, Willan AR, Wiececk EM, Taylor DR, Flannesy EM *et al.* A longitudinal, population-based cohort study of childhood asthma followed to adulthood. *The New England Journal of Medicine* 2003; 349(14): 1414–1422.

Stern DA, Morgan WJ, Halonen M, Wright AL, Martinez FD. Wheezing and bronchial hyper-responsiveness in early childhood as predictors of newly diagnosed asthma in early adulthood: a longitudinal birth-cohort study. *Lancet* 2008; 372: 1058–1064.

Further reading

Bateman ED, Hurd SS, Barnes PJ *et al.* Global strategy for asthma management and prevention: GINA executive summary. *The European Respiratory Journal* 2008; 31: 143–178.

British Thoracic Society and the Scottish Intercollegiate Guidelines Network British Guideline on the Management of Asthma. *Thorax* 2008; 63 (supplement IV).

Bucknell CE, Slack R, Godley CC, Mackay TW, Wright SC. Scottish Confidential Inquiry in to Asthma Deaths (SCIAD) 1994–1996. *Thorax* 2000; 54: 978–984.

O'Byrne PM, Pedersen S, Lamm CJ, Tan WC, Busse WW; START Investigators Group. Severe exacerbations and decline in lung function in asthma. *American Journal of Respiratory and Critical Care Medicine* 2009; 179: 19–24.

Taylor DR, Bateman ED, Boulet L-P *et al.* A new perspective on concepts of asthma severity and control. *The European Respiratory Journal* 2008; 32: 546–554.

CHAPTER 5

Precipitating Factors

John Rees

Sherman Education Centre, Guy's Hospital, London, UK

> **OVERVIEW**
>
> - Airways in asthmatic patients are usually sensitive to non-specific stimuli, such as dust and smoke, as well as respond to specific agents
> - Exercise often provokes asthma but does not increase bronchial responsiveness. Asthmatics should be encouraged to take treatment to maintain regular exercise
> - House dust mite provides the commonest positive skin test in the United Kingdom, but attempts to reduce the exposure produce little benefit
> - Food allergy causes eczema and gastrointestinal symptoms more often than asthma, but some striking cases do occur
> - Occupational exposure is an important factor in up to 10% cases of adult asthma
> - Most asthma drugs can be used safely in pregnancy

Bronchial hyper-responsiveness

The concept of increased reactivity of the airway to specific and non-specific stimuli is discussed in Chapter 2. While inflammatory change in the airway wall is associated with increased reactivity, the underlying mechanisms of increased bronchial reactivity are uncertain (Figure 5.1). The sustained reactivity found in asthmatic patients has been attributed to imbalance of autonomic control or other non-adrenergic, non-cholinergic plexuses, abnormal immunological and cellular responses, increased permeability of the epithelium and intrinsic differences in the action of smooth muscle or its hypertrophy.

Non-specific stimuli

Airways in asthmatic patients are usually sensitive to non-specific stimuli such as dust and smoke. Laughing or coughing may provoke wheezing. Specific responses to agents such as pollen may lead to increased non-specific reactivity and symptoms of asthma for days or even weeks. Upper respiratory viral infections may lead to similar changes and may increase reactivity in non-asthmatic

subjects. In contrast, avoidance of exposure to known allergens may lead to improved control of asthma with reduced responses to other stimuli. Challenge to airways by specific allergens may induce late responses 6 to 10 hours after exposure. Such late responses may mimic more closely the inflammatory changes caused by asthma that occur spontaneously. They lead to a subsequent rise in non-specific airway reactivity.

Exercise

Vigorous exercise produces narrowing of the airways in most asthmatic patients and, as described in Chapter 2, can be used as a simple diagnostic test. Asthma during or after exercise is most likely to be a practical problem in children, where it may interfere with games at school. The type of exercise influences the response; most asthmatic patients find that swimming in warm indoor pools is the activity least likely to induce an attack. This observation has been explained by clinical studies showing the importance of cooling and drying of the airways during hyperventilation and exercise. The effect of exercise can be mimicked by breathing cold, dry air, whereas breathing warm, humid air – as in indoor swimming pools – prevents the asthmatic response (Figure 5.2). In some patients, however, this picture is confusing, because they are sensitive to the chemical agents used in swimming pools.

Drug prophylaxis

Protection against exercise-induced asthma is provided by many of the commonly used drugs. Use of a short-acting β-agonist 15 to

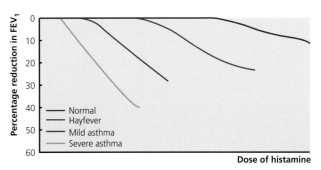

Figure 5.1 Bronchial reactivity is increased in people with asthma, particularly in those with severe disease.

ABC of Asthma, 6th edition. By J. Rees, D. Kanabar and S. Pattani.
Published 2010 by Blackwell Publishing.

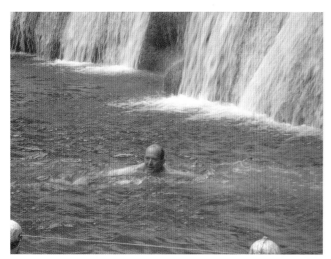

Figure 5.2 Swimming is the exercise least likely to provoke exercise-induced asthma.

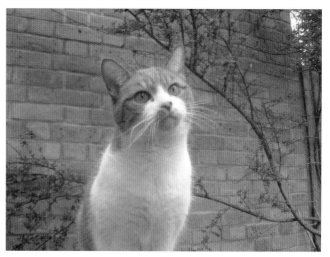

Figure 5.3 Cats are the most problematic domestic pet for people with asthma.

30 minutes before exercise is usually effective and such treatments will normally allow a child to take part in games at school. Sodium cromoglicate and nedocromil sodium also block the response. Long-acting β-agonists and leukotriene receptor antagonists are effective in preventing or minimising exercise-induced asthma. It may be necessary to explain to teachers the use of drugs and the objectives of the treatment.

Exercise itself is unlikely to have any major beneficial effect on asthma, but general fitness and weight control should be encouraged. A fit person can do a given task with less overall ventilation than an unfit one – hence the reduced likelihood of exercise-induced asthma. Asthma is quite compatible with a successful sporting career, as a number of athletes have testified, and the common inhaled asthma drugs are allowed in the regulations of most sporting bodies including inhaled corticosteroids and long-acting β-agonists. The need for medication should be declared in advance. The number of athletes using asthmatic medication has increased and the International Olympic Committee requires medical confirmation and may require on-site testing to show the need for medication. Various over-the-counter preparations for upper airway symptoms are not allowed.

Refractoriness

A second bout of exercise within an hour or so of the first is often less troublesome, a phenomenon known as *refractoriness*. The general benefits of warming up before exercise may therefore be increased for asthmatic athletes. Late asthmatic responses 4 to 6 hours after exposure are common after exposure to allergens, but they are rare and not troublesome after exercise.

Allergens at home

Pets

The parents of asthmatic children often worry about household pets. Cats cause the greatest problem, with allergens in saliva, urine and dander, but most domestic animals can trigger asthma on occasions. Associated symptoms of conjunctivitis and rhinitis are very common. Patients who have major problems with their asthma should be advised not to acquire any new pets (Figure 5.3).

Animal allergens remain in the house long after the pet is removed and so, if problems are suspected, the pet should move out for a month or two; alternatively the patient could move out for a week or two. Unjustified removal of favourite pets without good reason may, however, provoke more serious problems from emotional upset.

However, the position is complicated by evidence that exposure to cats and dogs in early life may result in a lower prevalence of asthma. It may be that early exposure helps in maturation of the immune system and the switch to a Th2 lymphocyte phenotype, the 'hygiene' hypothesis.

Dust mites

The house dust mite, *Dermatophagoides pteronyssinus*, provides the material for the most common positive skin prick test in the United Kingdom (Figure 5.4). The main allergen is found in the mites' faecal pellets. The mites live off human skin scales; are widely distributed in bedding, furniture, carpets and soft toys; and thrive best in warm, damp conditions. The expectation of a warm environment at home has increased the exposure of children to allergens and is likely to be an element contributing to the increased prevalence of asthma.

Change of environment

It patients move into environments that are completely free of house dust mites their symptoms improve. This can be achieved in the mountains of Switzerland or near home but in less picturesque surroundings, in specially cleaned hospital wards without soft furnishings.

It is much more difficult to reduce the numbers of mites sufficiently at home. Regular cleaning of bedrooms and avoiding

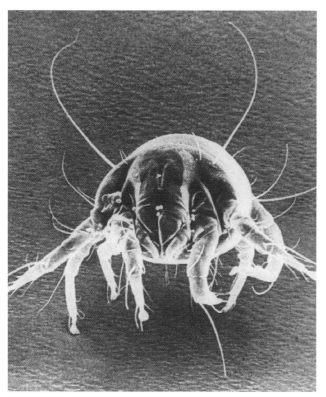

Figure 5.4 Dust mite.

materials that are particularly likely to collect dust are sensible measures to keep down the antigenic load (Box 5.1).

Box 5.1 **Measures to control house dust mites**

Though the effects are small, families who want to deal with house dust mites can try the following:

- Impervious covers on mattresses and soft furnishings
- Hard floors instead of carpets
- No soft toys in the bedroom
- Acaricides applied regularly to soft furnishings
- Washing bed clothes at high temperatures
- Damp dusting
- Dehumidification

Substantial reduction in mite antigen is possible by reducing the use of soft furnishing and carpets, extensive cleaning and the use of mattress covers made of materials such as Gortex, which are impermeable to mites. Acaricides, or even applications of liquid nitrogen to mattresses, can produce a temporary drop. Vacuum cleaners fitted with fine filters may help, in combination with measures that address reservoirs of antigen in sites such as mattresses. Although these measures reduce mite numbers, they have little effect on asthma control probably because they do not produce enough of a sustained reduction in house dust mite antigen (Gotzsche *et al.*, 2004). Families may want to reduce mite exposure but it cannot be recommended as a useful, cost-effective strategy based on current evidence.

Cockroaches

In some areas asthmatics show high levels of sensitivity to cockroach allergen. These levels can be around 50% in institutions and lower socio-economic groups.

Diet

Food allergy causes eczema and gastrointestinal symptoms more often than asthma, but some striking cases of asthma do occur. Exclusion diets have generally given disappointing results in asthma; immediate skin prick tests and radio-allergosorbent tests are less useful than for inhaled allergens. Most serious cases of asthma induced by food intolerance are evident from a carefully taken history, so elaborate diets are not warranted. When there is doubt, suspicions can be confirmed by excluding the agent from the diet or by controlled exposure.

Intolerance to food does not always indicate an allergic mechanism. Reactions may be related to pharmacological mediators such as histamine or tyramine in the food. They may be produced by food additives such as the yellow dye tartrazine, which is added to a wide range of foods and medications. When there is a specific allergy to foodstuffs, the most likely to be implicated are milk, eggs, nuts and wheat. Management can be difficult because of the use of nuts in a wide range or products.

Diets low in antioxidants such as vitamin C, vitamin E and selenium (meat, fish and nuts) are associated with asthma. Supplementation has not been shown to be effective but a good mixed diet with adequate quantities of vitamin C (fruit and vegetables) and vitamin E (plant oils, nuts and cereals) should be encouraged.

Pollens and spores

Seasonal asthma, often together with rhinitis and conjunctivitis, is most usually associated with grass pollens, which are most common during June and July (Figure 5.5). Less common in the United Kingdom is precipitation of asthma by tree pollens, many of which are produced between February and May and mould spores from Cladosporium and Alternaria, which abound in July

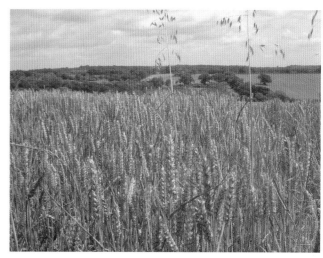

Figure 5.5 Exposure to specific pollens and spores can be seasonal.

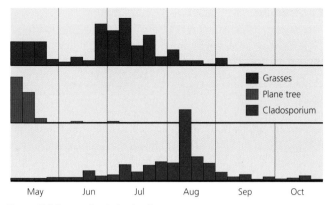

Figure 5.6 Seasonal variation in allergens.

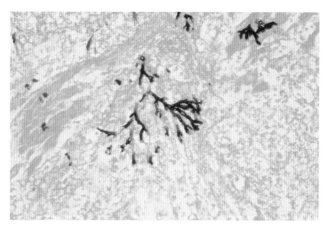

Figure 5.8 *Aspergillus fumigatus* hyphae and conidiiophores (fruiting heads).

and August (Figure 5.6). Complete avoidance of such widespread pollens is impractical. A number of studies show some benefit of immunotherapy and advances in allergen production, and their manipulation may lead to greater use of this therapy in future.

In most patients, immunotherapy is unnecessary because inhaled drugs provide adequate control and are simple to use. The strong placebo effect, allergic reactions to hyposensitisation and the occasional mortality must also be taken into account in assessing its value. Systematic reviews have shown that symptoms and bronchial responsiveness can be reduced by specific immunotherapy, and the sublingual route may provide a safer, simpler option in the future.

Allergic bronchopulmonary aspergillosis

Some asthmatic patients develop sensitivity to the spores of *Aspergillus fumigatus*, which is a common fungus particularly

partial to rotting vegetation. Allergic bronchopulmonary aspergillosis is associated with eosinophilia in blood and sputum, rubbery brownish plugs of mucus containing fungal hyphae and proximal bronchiectasis. Areas of consolidation and collapse may be visible in the chest X-ray film and each episode can lead to further bronchiectatic damage (Figures 5.7 and 5.8). The aspergillus skin test will be positive and specific immunoglobulin E (IgE) will be found in the blood.

Individual episodes settle after treatment with corticosteroids but if they are frequent and bronchiectasis is developing then long-term oral corticosteroids may be appropriate. Antifungal imidazoles such as itraconazole may also reduce the frequency of attack (Wark, 2004).

Occupational asthma

The importance of occupational asthma is increasingly being recognised. Some estimates suggest that at least 10% of cases of adult onset or relapsing asthma have an occupational component and over 400 precipitating agents have been reported (Box 5.2). Although asthmatic patients choosing a career should avoid occupations where they are likely to be exposed to large quantities of non-specific stimuli such as dust and cold air, previous asthma is not a reliable predictor of occupational asthma. An occupational element should always be considered, particularly with adult onset asthma (Figure 5.9). The commonest reported occupations are as paint sprayers, bakers, nurses, chemical workers and animal handlers.

Box 5.2 **Some causes of occupational asthma**

Chemicals

- Isocyanates
- Platinum salts
- Epoxy resins
- Aluminium
- Hair sprays
- Azodicarbonamide (plastic blowing)

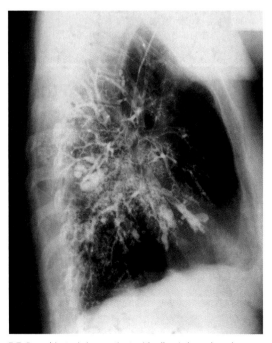

Figure 5.7 Bronchiectasis in a patient with allergic bronchopulmonary aspergillosis.

Vegetable sources

- Wood dusts
- Dust metal such as flour from grains
- Coffee beans
- Colophony (solders)
- Cotton, flax, hemp, dust
- Castor bean dust
- Latex

Enzymes

- Trypsin
- *Bacillus subtilis*

Animals

- Laboratory rodents
- Shellfish
- Larger mammals
- Locusts
- Grain weevil, mites

Drug manufacture

- Penicillins
- Piperazine
- Salbutamol
- Cimetidine
- Isphaghula
- Ipecacuanha

Definition

Occupational asthma is officially recognised as an industrial disease and subject to compensation. It is defined as asthma that 'develops after a variable period of symptomless exposure to a sensitising agent at work' (www.occupationalasthma.com). The UK Health and Safety Executive website lists nearly 50 agents recognised as causes of occupational asthma (http://www.hse.gov.uk/asthma/substances.htm). Agents such as proteolytic enzymes and laboratory animals are particularly likely to produce problems in atopic subjects, whereas isocyanate asthma is not related to atopic status. In some studies, potent agents such as platinum salts have produced asthma in up to half of those who are exposed to them.

Diagnosis

When occupational asthma is considered, questions should be asked about the relation between symptoms and time at and away from work. Increased bronchial reactivity provoked by occupational agents may persist long after removal from exposure. Regular peak flow recordings are once again an important diagnostic tool and usually show a distinct relation to time at work, but the relationship may not be obvious because the timing of the responses is variable. Reactions may occur soon after arriving at work, be delayed until later in the day or come on slowly over several days. In some cases, a weekend away from work may not be long enough for lung function to return to normal and absence for a week

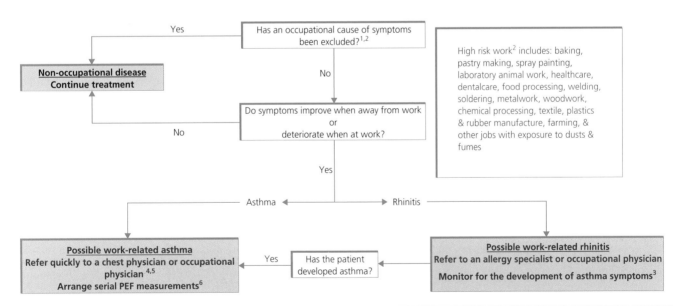

1. At least 1 in 10 cases of new or recurrent asthma in adult life are attributable to occupation.
2. Enquire of adult patients with rhinitis or asthma about their job and the materials with which they work.
3. Rhino-conjunctivitis may precede IgE-associated occupational asthma; the risk of developing asthma being highest in the year after the onset of rhinitis.
4. The prognosis of occupational asthma is improved by early identification and early avoidance of further exposure to its cause.
5. Confirm a diagnosis supported by objective criteria and not on the basis of a compatible history alone because of the potential implications for employment.
6. Arrange for workers whom you suspect of having work-related asthma to perform serial peak flow measurements at least four times a day.

Figure 5.9 Work-related asthma and rhinitis: case finding and management in primary care (from 'Guidelines for the Identification, Management & Prevention of Occupational Asthma', British Occupational Heath Research Foundation).

or two may be necessary. Initial investigations include exploring potential agents at work and recording peak flow patterns every 2 or 4 hours at and away from work. A computer programme exists to analyse peak flow recordings in suspected occupational asthma (http://www.occupationalasthma.com). Further investigation may require specific challenge testing in an experienced laboratory. There are few useful standardised immunological tests.

Management

Awareness and early detection are important since occupational asthma is the one area where appropriate management can affect the natural history of the disease. Shorter duration and better lung function are associated with a better response to management and improvement or resolution of asthma is most likely in those who have no further exposure. If adjustment of conditions at work is not possible then a change of job may be necessary. It is advisable to try to obtain, with the patient's consent, the co-operation of any occupational health staff in the firm at an early stage. Employers are requested to report cases under the Reporting of Injuries, Diseases and Dangerous Occurrences Regulations (RIDDOR).

Drug-induced asthma

Two main groups of drugs are responsible for most cases of drug-induced asthma: β-blocking agents and prostaglandin synthetase inhibitors such as aspirin (Box 5.3).

Box 5.3 **Drugs that can induce asthma**

- β-blockers (including eye drops)
- Aspirin and non-steroidal anti-inflammatory drugs
- Inhaled asthma drugs
- Nebuliser solutions, hypotonic or with preservatives
- Angiotensin-converting enzyme inhibitors

β-blockers

β-blocking agents usually induce bronchoconstriction when given to asthmatic patients and this may happen even when they are given in eye drops (Figure 5.10). Relatively selective β-blockers such as atenolol and metoprolol are less likely to cause severe irreversible asthma, but the whole group of β-blocking drugs should be avoided in patients who already have asthma. For hypertension diuretics, angiotensin-converting enzyme inhibitors, or calcium antagonists are suitable alternatives. When asthma is produced by β-blockade, large doses of β-stimulants are necessary to reverse it, particularly with less selective β-blockers. Fortunately, cardiac side-effects of treatment with β-stimulants are not a problem because they are also inhibited by the β-blockade.

Prostaglandin synthetase inhibitors

Salicylates provoke severe narrowing of the airways in a small group of adults with asthma; 2–3% of asthmatics have aspirin sensitivity on history taking, but around 20% have some sensitivity

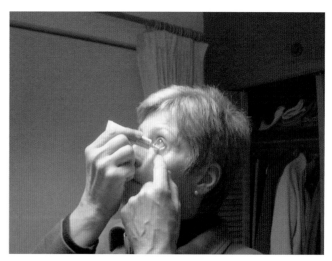

Figure 5.10 Absorption of β-blockers through the conjunctiva can precipitate asthma.

on provocation testing. Once such a reaction has been noted, these patients should avoid contact with aspirin or non-steroidal anti-inflammatory agents, which usually produce the same effects. The mechanism is probably related to changes in arachidonic acid metabolism with increased production of leukotrienes (Figure 5.11). Milder salicylate sensitivity can be shown more often on routine testing, particularly in adults with asthma and nasal polyps.

Ibuprofen is available without prescription and has the same effects. Patients are often unaware of the presence of salicylate in common compound preparations and cold cures. When salicylate sensitivity is suspected patients should be asked to check carefully the contents of any such medication they take. Apart from avoidance, aspirin-sensitive asthmatics are generally managed in the same way as those with other forms of asthma. It may be possible to induce tolerance to salicylates by carefully building up from small oral doses. This should be done only in experienced units.

Iatrogenic effects

Very occasionally drugs used to treat asthma can themselves be responsible for provoking bronchoconstriction. Such paradoxical

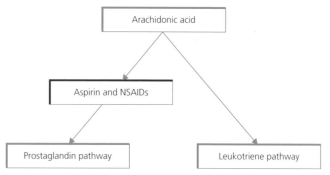

Figure 5.11 Aspirin blocks prostaglandin synthetase activity and sends arachidonic acid metabolism down the leukotriene pathway. This is likely to be the basis of aspirin-induced asthma.

effects have been described with aminophylline, ipratropium bromide, sodium cromoglycate, β-agonists in infants and propellants or contaminants from the valve apparatus in metered dose inhalers.

Hypotonic solutions are a potent cause of bronchoconstriction in people with asthma, and nebuliser solutions should be made up with normal saline rather than water. Preservatives in some nebuliser solutions have also produced narrowing of the airways.

Emotional factors

Psychological factors can play an important part in asthma. On their own they do not produce asthma in subjects without an underlying susceptibility, but in the laboratory emotional factors and expectation can influence the bronchoconstrictor responses to various specific and non-specific stimuli and the bronchodilator responses to treatment. Stress and emotional disturbance are factors that must be taken into account in the overall management of asthmatic patients. In children, the position is complicated by the emotional responses of their parents.

Confidence and relaxation

Emotional problems are more likely to occur when control of asthma is poor and these problems are best managed by increasing the confidence of patients and relatives with adequate explanation and control of the asthma. It is particularly important that patients know exactly what to do during an acute exacerbation. More specific measures such as relaxation, yoga, hypnotherapy and acupuncture have been investigated (Figure 5.12). Some trials have shown beneficial effects and some patients obtain considerable help from relaxation treatment. If conventional medicines are neglected when alternative approaches are adopted, however, it can be dangerous.

Asthma associated with emotional outbursts such as laughing and crying may be related to the response of the hyper-reactive airways to deep inspirations or to inhalation of cold, dry air rather than to the emotion itself. Manipulative patients may, of course, use a disease such as asthma for their own purposes just as they might use any other chronic disease.

Pollution

Personal air pollution with cigarette smoke worsens asthma; active and passive smoking provokes narrowing of the airways.

Air quality

There has been increased interest in environmental pollution in recent years. Though the inner city smogs disappeared after the introduction of the Clean Air Act 1956, high levels of ozone, sulphur dioxide, oxides of nitrogen and particulate matter develop in certain areas and in particular climatic conditions (Figure 5.13). Combinations of high temperature, humidity and heavy traffic can cause levels of these pollutants that are above the recommended guidelines of the World Health Organization. Increased symptoms and admissions have been linked to levels of nitrogen dioxide and sulphur dioxide – and, in some studies, ozone. High levels of small particulate matter are associated with increased mortality from cardio-respiratory diseases. Asthmatics should be aware of measures of air quality.

Weather

Climatic conditions such as pressure and humidity associated with thunderstorms can provoke asthma. The conditions may increase the concentrations of fungal and pollen spores at ground level as they are brought down from higher levels of the atmosphere. The spores rupture to produce particles of respirable size.

Indoor environment

Indoor pollution can also cause problems. Oxides of nitrogen are produced from heating and cooking. Formaldehyde and moulds and other biological compounds may occur in dwellings. Levels of nitrogen dioxide found in the home may increase airway responses to common allergens such as house dust mite, and the average UK citizen spends 85% to 90% of their time indoors.

Asthma and pregnancy

The control of asthma during pregnancy can change but the effect is variable (Figure 5.14). About a third of patients improve, a third

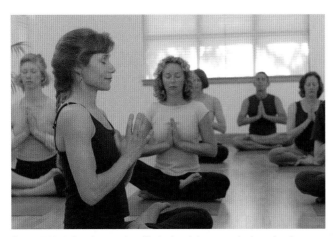

Figure 5.12 Relaxation can be of help, but it is not a substitute for drug therapy.

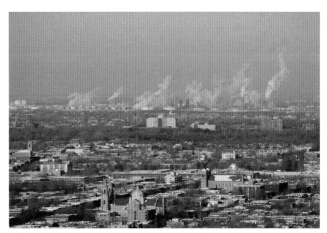

Figure 5.13 Air quality can be poor, especially in large cities.

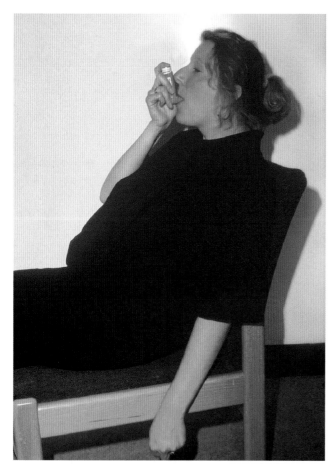

Figure 5.14 Inhaled drugs for asthma can be used normally during pregnancy without risk to the fetus.

worsen and a third continue unchanged. The effect may vary in different pregnancies in the same woman. Breathlessness may be more pronounced in late pregnancy as the diaphragmatic movement is limited even without any change in airflow obstruction.

Drug treatment during pregnancy

There is a natural anxiety about the use of drugs during pregnancy. Fortunately, the usual asthma treatments of inhaled β-agonists and inhaled and oral corticosteroids and theophyllines have been shown to be safe. Little information is available on leukotriene receptor antagonists. They should not be started in pregnancy but might be continued in patients who have shown a significant benefit. Asthma control and supervision should be improved during pregnancy to reduce the likelihood of an acute exacerbation. Acute attacks should be treated vigorously in the normal way. Severe asthma and hypoxia rather than asthma treatments are the potential danger during pregnancy. Treatment should be continued as usual through breastfeeding.

References

Gotzsche P, Johansen H, Schmidt L, Burr M. House dust mite control measures for asthma. *Cochrane Database System Review* 2004; 4: CD001187.

Wark P. Pathogenesis of allergic bronchopulmonary aspergillosis and an evidence based review of azoles in treatment. *Respiratory Medicine* 2004; 98: 915–923.

Further reading

Gannon PF, Newton DT, Belcher J, Pantin CF, Burge PS. Development of OASYS-2: a system for the analysis of serial measurement of peak expiratory flow in workers with suspected occupational asthma. *Thorax* 1996; 51: 484–489.

CHAPTER 6

General Management of Chronic Asthma

John Rees

Sherman Education Centre, Guy's Hospital, London, UK

OVERVIEW

- The asthma guidelines produced by the British Thoracic Society, the Scottish Intercollegiate Guidelines Network and others are used widely and are updated regularly
- Guidelines are most likely to influence behaviour when they are adapted to local needs and promoted by a local respected enthusiast
- Hospitals and practices should carry out regular audit against the agreed parts of the guidelines
- A major goal of asthma management is freedom from symptoms rather than tolerance of shortness of breath and frequent need of bronchodilators
- Goals and management plans should be discussed and agreed on with individual patients

Guidelines

Various guidelines have been produced and published for the management of asthma. In the United Kingdom those produced by the British Thoracic Society and the Scottish Intercollegiate Guidelines Network with Asthma UK, the Royal College of Physicians, the College of Emergency Medicine, NHS Quality Improvement Scotland and the General Practice Airways Group are used widely and form the basis of the recommendations in the book, the *ABC of Asthma* (*British guideline on the management of asthma*, 2008). They were first published in 2003, revised in 2008 and are updated annually. The Global Initiative for Asthma (GINA, http://www. ginasthma.com/) produces valuable guidelines and resources.

Guidelines are most likely to influence behaviour when they are adapted to local needs in hospital or practice and endorsed by a local respected enthusiast. They should be accompanied by regular audit against the agreed parts of the guidelines. Most of the published guidelines are in broad agreement on the strategy for managing chronic asthma.

In the United Kingdom, the general practitioner contract allows practices to earn points related to organisation of asthma management.

General features

As a preliminary step in all patients with asthma, obvious precipitating factors should be sought and avoided when practicable. This is possible for specific allergens such as animals and foods, but is not usually feasible with more widespread allergens such as pollens and house dust mites. A common non-specific stimulus is cigarette smoking. Up to a fifth of asthmatics continue to smoke; strenuous efforts should be made to discourage smoking in asthmatic patients and their families. Precipitating factors should be carefully explored on one of the first visits but they should also be reassessed periodically.

Patients with asthma often look for a cure. It is important to establish early on that cure is not possible but if patients accept the need for regular treatment most patients can be virtually free of symptoms.

Fortunately, most patients can achieve such control by safe drug treatment, with minimal or no side effects. Unfortunately, many patients with mild asthma fail to achieve this degree of control. Educating the patient in understanding the disease and treatment is often helped by home peak flow recording and written explanations of the purpose and practical details of treatment. In particular, the differences between symptomatic bronchodilator treatment and regular maintenance treatment must be emphasised. It is still not uncommon to find asthmatic patients using their dose of inhaled steroid only to treat an acute attack. In general practice and in hospital, nurses provide a vital element in the management of asthma.

Patients need to be involved in developing their asthma management plans. Their beliefs and goals need to be taken into account in producing a jointly agreed plan. Understanding of management plans, inhaler technique and adherence to plans should be checked regularly, particularly when control is not adequate and stepping up treatment is being considered.

Asthma clinics

Many hospitals have concentrated their patients into specific asthma clinics for some years. Many general practices have specific asthma or respiratory disease clinics run by practice nurses. Others use the nurses in clinics for other chronic conditions as well as asthma. Local and national training courses are available for

ABC of Asthma, 6th edition. By J. Rees, D. Kanabar and S. Pattani.
Published 2010 by Blackwell Publishing.

nurses who take on such clinics, for example, Education for Health (http://www.educationforhealth.org.uk/ formerly the National Respiratory Training Centre) in Warwick. The clinics can be used to audit the treatment of asthmatic patients in a practice and to ensure that all patients are encouraged to participate in their optimal management.

Asthma clinics in general practice are best if they work with clearly written management guidelines and care plans. In some practices they are run by doctors, but in most cases they are run by nurses, who have more time to spend with each individual patient to go through inhaler techniques and understand their management plans. An interested doctor should be available for consultation and a close liaison should be built up with chest physicians at the local hospital. Every patient should have a personal management plan and be reviewed at least once a year and the clinic should be subject to regular audit.

Aims of management

Persistent inflammation of the airways and increased bronchial reactivity have been recognised even in mild intermittent asthma.

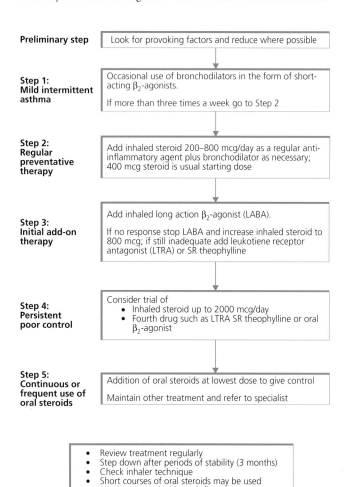

Figure 6.1 Stepwise treatment of asthma (adapted from guidelines from the British Thoracic Society and Scottish Intercollegiate Guidelines Network). The inhaled steroid would be beclometasone dipropionate, budesonide or fluticasone propionate (starting at half the dose shown).

The inflammation can be targeted by drugs such as inhaled corticosteroids, which reduce bronchial hyper-responsiveness, symptoms and inflammatory infiltration of the airway. There has been a general move to be more aggressive in the treatment of asthma, the goal being freedom from symptoms rather than tolerance of shortness of breath and frequent need of bronchodilators (Figure 6.1). Once control is achieved, the regime is usually maintained for 3–6 months before stepping down the treatment.

Drug regimes

Routine regular use of short-acting bronchodilators should be avoided. They should be used to treat symptoms and their use should be limited by the use of prophylactic agents. This approach fits with the various sets of published guidelines (Box 6.1).

> Box 6.1 **Control of asthma**
>
> The *British Guideline on the Management of Asthma* was first produced by the British Thoracic Society (BTS) and Scottish Intercollegiate Guidelines Network (SIGN) in January 2003 and last updated in 2008. Updates appear regularly. They express the aim of asthma as control of the disease defined as follows, with minimal side effects:
>
> - No day-time symptoms
> - No night-time awakening due to asthma
> - No need for rescue medication
> - No exacerbations
> - No limitations on activity during exercise
> - Normal lung function (Forced expiratory volume in 1 second (FEV1) and/or peak expiratory flow (PEF) >80% predicted or best)
>
> At stages four to five such freedom from symptoms may not be achievable without side effects, and the objectives are as follows:
>
> - Fewest possible symptoms
> - Least possible need for relief bronchodilators
> - Least possible limitation of activity
> - Least possible PEF variation
> - Best PEF
> - Fewest adverse effects of treatment

Regular inhaled corticosteroids decrease reactivity, as do leukotriene receptor antagonists and (probably) sodium cromoglycate and nedocromil sodium. Studies of mild asthma show that regular use of prophylactic agents reduces inflammation of the airways and that inhaled steroids do this most effectively. The hope is that the reduction in the inflammation will prevent damage to the airway that would otherwise go on to produce irreversible obstruction (Figure 6.2). There is still no convincing long-term evidence for this, nor is there convincing evidence that inhaled steroids change the natural history of asthma in any other way. Reactivity is improved but does not return to normal and reverts to pre-treatment levels on stopping steroids. Leukotriene receptor antagonists have shown evidence of an anti-inflammatory action in addition to bronchodilatation.

Mild episodes of wheezing occurring once or twice a month can be controlled with inhaled β_2-agonists. When attacks are more

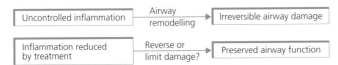

Figure 6.2 Control of inflammation in the airway wall may prevent or limit irreversible airway changes.

frequent, regular treatment with an inflammatory agent is necessary although inhaled corticosteroids have been used successfully as needed in a study of very mild asthma. Lack of adequate control should be sought by questions about sensitivity to irritants such as dust and smoke, questions about night-time symptoms and by peak flow recording. Definite diurnal variation on peak flow readings or nocturnal waking indicates a high degree of reactivity of the airways and the need for vigorous treatment. When chronic symptoms persist in the face of appropriate inhaled treatment, a short course of oral corticosteroids often produces improvement, which may last for many months after the course.

Long-acting inhaled β_2-agonists are good at controlling symptoms. They do not have a significant effect on underlying inflammation and should only be used in combination with inhaled steroids. Used alone they may be associated with increased mortality and morbidity. In view of this it seems sensible to use them in a combined preparation.

In a variable disease such as asthma, in which monitoring of the state of the disease is comparatively easy, the education and co-operation of the patient are vital parts of management. The patient should know how and when to take each treatment, broadly what each does and exactly what to do in an exacerbation. These should be set out in a written plan specific for individual patients and produced in consultation with them.

References

British Thoracic Society and the Scottish Intercollegiate Guidelines Network British guideline on the management of asthma. http://www.brit-thoracic.org.uk/Portals/0/Clinical%20Information/Asthma/Guidelines/asthma_final2008.pdf. *Thorax* 2008; 63 (Suppl IV).

Global strategy for asthma management and prevention. Updated 2008; retrieved 17 November 2009 http://www.ginasthma.com/.

Further reading

Bateman ED, Hurd SS, Barnes PJ *et al.* Global strategy for asthma management and prevention. GINA executive summary. *The European Respiratory Journal* 2008; 131: 143–178.

Papi A, Canonica GW, Maestrelli P *et al.* BEST Study Group. Rescue use of beclomethasone and albuterol in a single inhaler for mild asthma. *The New England Journal of Medicine* 2007; 356: 2040–2052.

CHAPTER 7

Treatment of Chronic Asthma

John Rees

Sherman Education Centre, Guy's Hospital, London, UK

OVERVIEW

- The first line of treatment for relief of asthma is one of the selective β₂-agonists taken by inhalation
- Long-acting inhaled β-agonists should be evaluated as an addition to a low to moderate dose of inhaled corticosteroids when control is inadequate on inhaled corticosteroids alone
- Long-acting inhaled β-agonists should not be used alone in asthma
- Inhaled corticosteroids are the most effective preventative therapy in asthma
- Many asthmatic patients turn to alternative therapies in the management of their asthma but few have any proven value

β-agonists

The first line of treatment for relief of asthma is one of the selective β₂-agonists taken by inhalation (Figure 7.1). β₂-agonists are the most effective bronchodilators in asthma. They start to work quickly – salbutamol and terbutaline take effect within 15 minutes and last for 4 to 6 hours. There is no clear threshold for all patients, but if there has been an exacerbation of asthma in the last 2 years, inhaled β₂-agonists are needed or symptoms present at least three times a week or asthma disturbs sleep one night a week, then additional treatment must be considered. The dose response varies among patients as does the dose that will produce side effects, such as tremor. Patients should be taught to monitor their inhaler use and to understand that if they need it more, or if its effects lessen, these are danger signals. They indicate deterioration in asthmatic control and the need for further treatment.

Adverse effects

Some patients worry that β₂-agonists may become less effective with time, particularly if the dose is high. There is little evidence of clinically significant tachyphylaxis for the airway effects in asthmatics. If it exists, it is a minor effect that is quickly reversed, either by stopping the treatment temporarily or by taking corticosteroids. Tremor, palpitations and muscle cramps may occur, but are rarely

troublesome if the drug is inhaled; these adverse effects outside the lung often become less of a problem with continued treatment.

Some studies found that regular use of β₂-agonists was associated with increased bronchial reactivity, worsening asthma control and accelerated decline of lung function. These have not been confirmed. However, when the steps in standard guidelines are followed, β₂-agonists are not used regularly unless needed for control of symptoms and in this way never without a regular preventer therapy such as inhaled steroids.

Long-acting β-agonists

The long-acting inhaled β₂-agonists salmeterol and formoterol have taken an increasing role in treatment since the early 1990s (Figure 7.2). The mechanism of the prolonged action is different with the two drugs and the onset of bronchodilatation is faster with formoterol, but in other ways the two drugs are regarded as equivalent by most physicians. They are particularly effective for nocturnal asthma and for exercise-induced asthma.

The British guidelines now place them as first option at "step 3" when a low to moderate dose of inhaled corticosteroids (400–800 µg beclometasone or equivalent) fail to establish symptom free control.

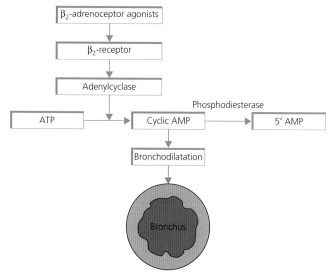

Figure 7.1 Increases in cyclic AMP lead to bronchodilatation and may be produced by β₂-receptor stimulation or phosphodiesterase inhibition.

ABC of Asthma, 6th edition. By J. Rees, D. Kanabar and S. Pattani.
Published 2010 by Blackwell Publishing.

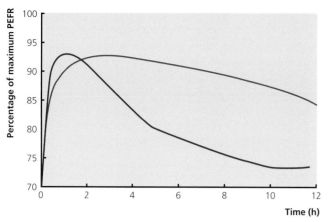

Figure 7.2 Bronchodilator response to inhaled salbutamol 200 μg (Violet line) and inhaled salmeterol 50 μg (Blue line). PEFR, Peak expiratory flow rate. Adapted from Ullman A *et al. Thorax* 1988; 4343: 674–678.

The response should be evaluated over 6–12 weeks. A minority of asthmatics show little or no benefit and, in them, the long-acting β-agonists (LABAs) should be stopped.

Several studies have shown that salmeterol is more effective than doubling inhaled corticosteroids in controlling symptoms and increasing peak flow (Pauwels *et al.*, 1997) (Figure 7.3). The effect is maintained over 6 months in such studies. A comparison of low- and high-dose inhaled steroids over 12 months, with or without formoterol, showed that increasing steroids and formoterol reduced exacerbations. Severe exacerbations, defined by need for oral steroids or peak flow drop, were prevented more effectively by higher dose steroids than formoterol, but best of all by the combination. Formoterol added to steroids was the most effective in symptom reduction and peak flow control. It is important to remember that the LABAs are bronchodilators and do not suppress inflammation. In asthma, they should always be given in combination with inhaled steroids and the patient must not drop these on starting or finding a highly effective medication. LABAs have been linked to increased mortality in asthma and the risk–benefit ratio should be considered and discussed. Any increased mortality may be limited to patients not taking simultaneous inhaled corticosteroids and balanced with the fact that LABAs are the most effective agent

for symptom control in those not controlled by low-dose inhaled corticosteroids.

Adverse effects of salmeterol and formoterol are the same as those of short-acting agents. Patients on LABAs should carry a short-acting β-agonist for immediate relief, although the fast onset of action of formoterol allows it to be used for regular dosing and acute relief, in combination with inhaled corticosteroids.

Anticholinergic bronchodilators

Ipratropium bromide blocks the cholinergic bronchoconstrictor effect of the vagus nerve (Figure 7.4). It is a non-selective antagonist blocking inhibitory M2 receptors on postganglionic nerves as well as M3 receptors on airway smooth muscle. A longer acting agent tiotropium is available for chronic obstructive pulmonary disease (COPD).

Effectiveness

Anticholinergics are most effective in very young children and in older patients. They are as effective as, or more effective than, β2-agonists in COPD. In asthma, anticholinergic agents are less effective than β2-agonists, but they may be tried as a supplement to β-agonists if reversibility is incomplete. Anticholinergics may be useful in the few patients who experience troublesome tremor or tachycardia.

Methylxanthines

Theophylline is an effective bronchodilator and may also have some anti-inflammatory actions. Its safety margin is low compared to other bronchodilators that can be given by inhalation (Figure 7.5).

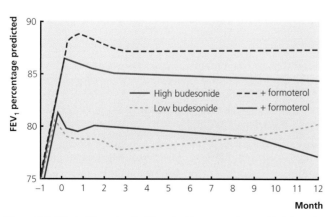

Figure 7.3 Effect of formoterol with and without a corticosteroid. Adapted from Pauwels RA *et al. The New England Journal of Medicine* 1997; 337: 1405–1411. Copyright © *1997 Massachusetts Medical Society. All rights reserved.*

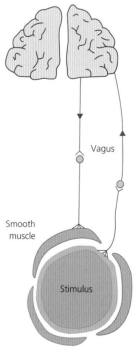

Figure 7.4 Anticholinergic agents block vagal efferent stimulation of bronchial smooth muscle.

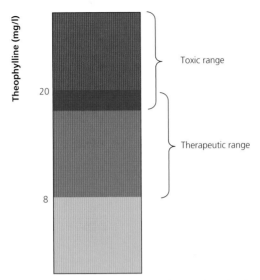

Figure 7.5 There is no safety margin between therapeutic and toxic ranges with theophylline.

Individual differences in the doses required are high and so it is necessary to monitor treatment through blood concentrations. Inhaled treatment with β-agonists is preferable, but slow-release theophyllines can be used as an alternative to long-acting β-agonists for nocturnal symptoms.

Adverse effects

The most common side effects of theophylline are nausea, vomiting and abdominal discomfort, but headache, malaise, fast pulse rate and fits also occur, sometimes without early warning from gastrointestinal symptoms (Box 7.1). The dose of theophylline should start at around 7 mg/kg/day in divided doses and should then be built up. All patients taking theophylline should have their serum concentrations monitored and doses adjusted until they are between 8 and 18 mg/l (40–90 μmol/l) for optimal bronchodilator effect. Above 20 mg/l toxic effects are unacceptably high, although gastrointestinal effects are common at lower concentrations. Absorption rates vary with long-acting preparations and the same brand should be used in any individual.

> Box 7.1 **Side effects of theophylline**
>
> The following are the most common side effects of theophylline:
>
> - Nausea
> - Vomiting
> - Abdominal discomfort
>
> However, the following side effects can occur, sometimes without early warning from gastrointestinal symptoms:
>
> - Headache
> - Malaise
> - Fast pulse rate
> - Fits

Theophylline clearance is increased by smoking, alcohol consumption and enzyme-inducing drugs such as phenytoin, rifampicin and barbiturates. Clearance will be decreased and blood concentrations will rise if it is given at the same time as cimetidine, ciprofloxacin or erythromycin and in the presence of heart failure, liver impairment or pneumonia.

Lower theophylline levels, with a lower risk of side effects, have been shown to have an anti-inflammatory effect *in vivo* and *in vitro* but are less effective than inhaled corticosteroids.

Mast cell stabilisers

Sodium cromoglycate

Sodium cromoglycate blocks bronchoconstrictor responses to challenge by exercise and antigens. The original proposed mechanism of stabilisation of mast cells may not be the main mechanism of its action in asthma. Sodium cromoglycate is less effective than inhaled corticosteroids. With the introduction of leukotriene receptor antagonists there is little reason to prescribe cromoglycate.

Other mast cell stabilisers have been disappointing, possibly because of the additional effects of cromoglycate. The oral agent ketotifen produces drowsiness in 10% of patients and has little activity although used in some countries.

Nedocromil sodium

Nedocromil sodium has the same properties as sodium cromoglycate but may have an additional anti-inflammatory effect on the airway epithelium and reduce coughing. However, there is still very little reason to consider it unless patients will not take inhaled steroids.

Inhaled corticosteroids

Inhaled corticosteroids form the most effective preventative therapy in asthma. Steroids may be given by metered dose inhaler, dry powder devices or nebuliser and the dose should be adjusted to give optimum control. Two common inhaled steroids, beclometasone dipropionate and budesonide, are roughly equivalent in dose, while fluticasone and mometasone have the same effect at half the dose.

Method of delivery

The formulation and delivery device must also be considered. The non-chlorofluorocarbon (CFC) beclometasone metered dose inhaler QVar has a small particle size and increased lung deposition (Leach, 1998) (Figure 7.6). The dose of beclometasone can be halved when switching from another preparation. Much of the benefit of inhaled corticosteroids is seen at low to moderate doses up to 400–800 μg of beclometasone. Further effect can be seen with higher doses but the dose response above 800 μg beclometasone or 500 μg fluticasone becomes flatter (Holt *et al.*, 2001).

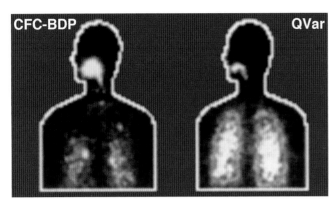

Figure 7.6 Deposition of beclometasone dipropionate after use of a standard metered dose inhaler and the CFC free Qvar inhaler (from Leach CL, *Respiratory Medicine* 1998; 92 (Suppl A0): 3–8). The latter produces a substantial increase in lung deposition (3M Healthcare).

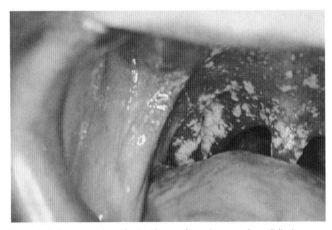

Figure 7.7 Spacers reduce the incidence of oropharyngeal candidiasis seen with inhaled corticosteroids.

Adverse effects

In adults, there are no problems apart from occasional oropharyngeal candidiasis (Figure 7.7) or a husky or weak voice (dysphonia) until a daily dose above the equivalent of 1000 μg beclometasone dipropionate is reached. At higher doses, there may be biochemical evidence of suppression of the hypothalamic–pituitary–adrenal axis, even with inhaled steroids (Table 7.1). Much of the systemic effect comes from absorption from the lung itself, bypassing the metabolic pathways of the gut and liver that limit any problems from drug deposited in the mouth and swallowed.

With doses of more than 1000 μg daily of budesonide or beclometasone there are identifiable metabolic effects. There is an

Table 7.1 Side effects of inhaled corticosteroids.

Established	Suggested at high dose
• Oropharyngeal candidiasis	• Irritation and cough
• Dysphonia	• Adrenal suppression
• Irritation and cough	• Reduced growth in children
Rare	• Osteoporosis
• Purpura and thinning of skin	
• Cataracts	

Table 7.2 Available inhaled corticosteroids.

Drug	Metered dose inhaler	Dry powder inhaler	Nebuliser	Combined with long-acting β-agonist
Beclometasone	+	+		+
Budesonide	+	+	+	+
Ciclesonide	+			
Fluticasone	+	+	+	+
Mometasone		+		

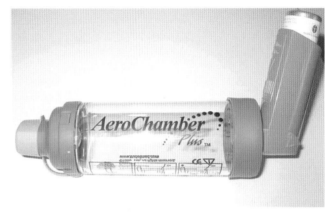

Figure 7.8 Large volume spacers overcome problems with coordination of inhaler firing and inspiration. They reduce oropharyngeal deposition of the aerosol and improve delivery to the lungs. A smaller volume spacer such as the one above is more convenient and seems to be as efficient as larger volume chambers (reproduced with permission from GlaxoSmithKline).

increase in the concentration of osteocalcin, a marker of increased bone turnover, but no evidence of clinical osteoporosis or fractures. There is some evidence of skin thinning and purpura, even in patients who have not had appreciable doses of oral steroids. Doses over 2000 μg daily are not often used but when necessary nebulised budesonide or fluticasone may be a convenient strategy. Ciclesonide may be less likely to produce effects on the hypothalamic–pituitary–adrenal axis (Table 7.2). At doses of >800 μg daily a spacer should be used to reduce pharyngeal deposition (Figure 7.8). At doses ≥1000 μg it has been suggested that patients should carry a steroid card, especially if they use regular courses of oral steroids.

Regular use

Doses of inhaled steroids should be taken regularly to be effective. Twice daily use is the usual frequency. In milder asthma under good control once daily use may be adequate and in very mild asthma, the use of therapy only as required has been successful. Doubling the regular dose when an upper respiratory infection develops has not been shown to have any benefit.

Adherence

The main difficulties in the use of inhaled corticosteroids are the patients' worries about the use of steroids and the difficulties of ensuring that patients take regular medication even when they are well. These problems may be increased by the move to use inhaled corticosteroids earlier in asthma and to achieve total asthma control free of symptoms. Combination with long-acting bronchodilators may improve adherence since loss of bronchodilator effect will be noticed more quickly.

Dosage reduction

There appears to be no advantage in starting a high dose to achieve quicker control. The starting dose should match the severity of the asthma and moderate levels are usually adequate and appropriate.

When asthma is under control the next decision is how long to maintain the inhaled steroids. The dose should be reviewed regularly, particularly at doses above 1000 μg daily. When aiming for complete control, this should be maintained for 3 months before reducing the inhaled steroid dose by 25–50%. Flexible regimens using formoterol and budesonide for regular and as needed use have been successful in establishing control and limiting steroid dosage. Regimes based on measures of inflammation (sputum eosinophilia) rather than symptoms have also shown better control at a lower total steroid dose.

Oral corticosteroids

Short courses of oral steroids are often necessary for acute exacerbations of asthma and have few serious problems. Occasional asthmatic patients have to take long-term oral corticosteroids, but this should be only after the failure of vigorous treatment with other drugs. The symptoms or risks of the disease must be balanced against the adverse effects of long-term treatment with oral corticosteroids (Figure 7.9).

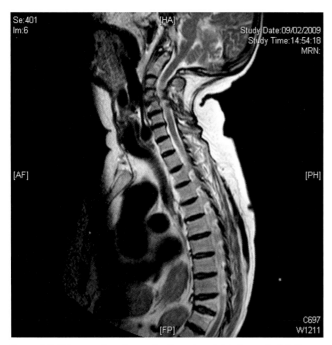

Figure 7.9 Osteoporotic collapse of a thoracic vertebra in a patient taking oral steroids.

Length of treatment

Short courses of oral steroids may be stopped abruptly or tailed off over a few days. Low concentrations of cortisol and adreno-corticotrophic hormone (ACTH) are found for just 2 to 3 days after 40 mg prednisolone daily for 3 weeks, but clinical problems with responses to stress or exacerbations of asthma do not occur. An appropriate course would be 30 to 50 mg prednisolone daily for a minimum of 5 days, usually up to 14 days until baseline function returns. Most asthmatic patients can be taught to keep such a supply of steroids at home and to use them according to their individual management plan when predetermined signs of deteriorating control occur.

If patients require long-term oral steroids, they should be settled on a regime of treatment on alternate days whenever possible. The goal is always to establish control with other treatment that will allow the discontinuation of the oral steroids. Inhaled steroids in moderate to high doses should be maintained to keep the oral dose as low as possible. Alternative preparations such as ACTH and triamcinolone are less flexible and give no appreciable benefit in terms of adrenal suppression.

Resistance

A small proportion of asthmatic patients are fully or partially resistant to corticosteroids. They form a particularly difficult group to treat but should be identified to avoid unnecessary, excessive steroid use.

Adverse effects

When patients are on long-term oral steroids or take short courses more than three times a year the risks of osteoporosis should be considered. Patients at high risk, such as those over 65 years, should start prophylactic treatment when they start regular steroids. Risk profiles can be calculated and treatment planned using templates from the National Osteoporosis Guideline Group (http://www.shef.ac.uk/NOGG/index.html). Regular exercise and adequate dietary vitamin D and calcium intake should be addressed in all patients on oral steroids.

Patients on steroids should be advised to avoid contact with chickenpox and *Herpes zoster* while on therapy and for 3 months after prolonged use. Blood glucose and blood pressure should be monitored in those on regular oral steroids.

Combined preparations

Some fixed dose combinations are available for the treatment of asthma. Combinations of bronchodilators may be used when such treatment has been shown to be appropriate in drug and in dose. This is unusual in asthma.

Combinations of long-acting inhaled bronchodilators and corticosteroids are convenient in chronic stable asthma and may improve adherence. Combinations of formoterol and budesonide can be varied with the severity and symptoms, since formoterol doses can be varied over a reasonable range and the onset of action of formoterol is fast enough for use as a reliever. Salmeterol is restricted to a dose of 50 mcg twice daily. Combined preparations of salmeterol and fluticasone are used to attain more prolonged periods of complete asthma control before adjustment of the dose, rather than more frequent adjustments to symptoms, the technique used successfully with the formoterol–budesonide combination. Other combinations of long-acting β-agonists and inhaled steroids are likely to be produced.

Leukotriene antagonists

The cysteinyl leukotrienes LTC4, LTD4 and LTE4 are inflammatory mediators formed from arachidonic acid by the action of the enzyme 5-lipoxygenase. They produce bronchoconstriction, oedema, mucus secretion, eosinophil recruitment and inflammation in the airway. Drugs such as montelukast and zafirlukast act as competitive inhibitors of receptors on smooth muscle and elsewhere. The other potential target is inhibition of 5-lipoxygenase itself (Figure 7.10).

Leukotriene receptor antagonists are only available for oral use. They should be taken an hour or two before or after food. Side effects are rare. They have been associated with Churg–Strauss syndrome (allergic granulomatosis) but in most cases this appears to be unmasking of the underlying problem by the reduction in steroid treatment possible after addition of zafirlukast.

Leukotriene receptor antagonists have been used in a variety of situations – as alternatives to inhaled steroids in prevention, as an alternative to long-acting β-agonists and as an additional treatment when control is difficult. Overall the effects are less than those achieved with inhaled steroids (O'Byrne et al., 2005). Nevertheless, they may be useful in patients who are not prepared to take inhaled steroids or those who have adverse responses or in exercise- or aspirin-induced asthma.

There is evidence that leukotriene receptor antagonists can reduce exacerbations and allow reduction in inhaled steroid dose when used as additional therapy. Long-acting β-agonists are the treatment of choice in patients not controlled with low to moderate dose inhaled steroids. Leukotriene receptor antagonists may be useful where control is still not adequate or long-acting β-agonists have been ineffective. They have the benefit of being effective on associated rhinitis.

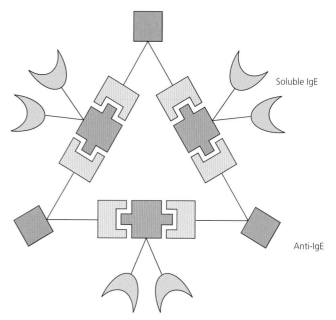

Figure 7.11 Anti-IgE binds to soluble IgE to form inactive hexamers and stops IgE cross linking and degranulating mast cells.

Anti-IgE monoclonal antibody

Monoclonal antibodies against immunoglobulin E (IgE) have been shown to be effective in asthma if IgE levels are reduced adequately (Figure 7.11). This is the first biotechnology therapy to be licensed for use in some countries. It has been shown to suppress early and late asthmatic reactions, reduce exacerbations and improve symptoms scores and to be steroid sparing in severe asthma. Current UK recommendations are for patients with allergies, on high-dose inhaled steroids and long-acting β-agonists, with impaired lung function and frequent exacerbations. Baseline IgE levels between 30 and 700 IU/ml and body weight determine the dose used. This is given by subcutaneous injection every 2 or 4 weeks, depending on the dose. Local reactions are common, usually but not always in the first 2 hours, and patients must be in a medically supervised environment with facilities for treatment of anaphylaxis. Treatment effectiveness is reviewed at 16 weeks.

Steroid-sparing agents

In patients requiring oral steroids to maintain control, a number of other agents have been used to try to reduce the steroid dose and avoid the associated side effects. All these treatments have side effects of their own and should be used under specialist advice with all other conventional therapies in place.

Methotrexate

There have been a number of trials of methotrexate, usually taken orally once a week. Around half of these have been positive with a significant reduction in steroid dose, and a trial of 2 to 3 months treatment may be appropriate in some patients. Adverse effects are on the bone marrow, liver and lung.

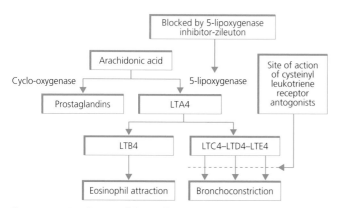

Figure 7.10 Site of action of drugs affecting the leukotriene system.

Other agents

Cyclosporin and oral gold have been effective in some studies, producing some improvement in control with a small decrease in steroid dose. Renal toxicity is a problem with both agents.

Reflux

Gastro-oesophageal reflux is often associated with asthma and should be treated appropriately, although it has been difficult to show a convincing benefit on asthma control.

Rhinitis

Rhinitis is a common accompaniment of asthma. It should be treated with nasal corticosteroids or a combined approach with leukotriene receptor antagonists.

Future treatments

Mediator antagonists are being investigated to follow on from the leukotriene receptor antagonists. Inhibition of Th2 cytokines such as anti-IL5 involved in eosinophil maturation and IL13 offer possibilities. Interference with Th1/Th2 balance might be possible but could have other immunological consequences. Other targets under study include antagonists of chemokines, adhesion molecules, tumour necrosis factor and inhibitors of phosphodiesterase type 4 (PDE-4 inhibitors).

Inhibitors of tryptase (a serine protease released from mast cells), nitric oxide production and kinases such as mitogen-activated protein kinase (MAPK) and Janus kinase (JAK) are other areas under active investigation. It is likely that the range of such treatments available will increase over the next few years.

Immunotherapy

Some patients have obvious precipitating factors – in particular, animals – and avoidance is helpful, but there are usually other unknown precipitating factors. More common are patients with reactive airways who are also sensitive to pollens, house dust mite and other allergens. Such stimuli are almost impossible to avoid completely in everyday life, although symptoms can improve with rigorous measures. Trials of subcutaneous desensitisation have produced limited benefit. Positive responses have been seen with desensitisation to house dust mite, grass pollen, tree pollen, cat and dog allergens and moulds.

Many asthmatic patients have multiple allergies, making immunotherapy less likely to be effective. The degree of control produced by desensitisation can often be achieved with simple, safe, inhaled drugs.

Newer techniques such as the sublingual route and peptide immunotherapy may provide tolerance, with a reduced likelihood of severe immune reactions.

There is little sound evidence to support desensitisation to other agents in asthmatic patients. In particular, cocktails produced from the results of skin or radioallergosorbent tests are not a valid form of treatment. Local reactions to desensitising agents are common and more generalised reactions and even death can occur. Most deaths have been related to errors in the injection schedule and inadequate supervision after injections. Desensitisation should be undertaken only where appropriate facilities for resuscitation are available.

Other challenges

One area where desensitisation is appropriate is in sensitivity to insect venom that results in anaphylaxis rather than asthma. Aspirin-induced asthma may respond to careful oral desensitisation.

Alternative treatments

Many asthmatic patients turn to alternative therapies in the management of their asthma. Most will use these alongside conventional therapies but may not inform their medical carers, particularly if they appear dismissive of such treatments. The dangers come when alternative treatments are used instead of standard treatments. Controlled trials are more difficult in this area and there are few examples of scientifically valid trials of adequate size and duration. Few of these techniques have been shown to have significant benefit in scientifically rigorous studies. However, it is best to work with patients who want to try these techniques, encouraging them to maintain conventional therapies alongside any other treatment.

Acupuncture

Control in trials is often adequate because the elements of treatment associated with the use of acupuncture needles make sham treatments difficult. Some short-term studies have shown some benefit on induced bronchoconstriction, but these do not compare with the effects of conventional pharmacological treatment. Some studies show that the acupuncture points are not important.

Relaxation, yoga and hypnotherapy

Various approaches have shown benefit in individual trials but none have been shown to be effective consistently in properly controlled studies. Hypnosis has been shown to have some effect, particularly in susceptible patients, as has pranayama yoga, a form of breathing control.

Breathing exercises

The Buteyko technique of breathing control has been promoted as an effective treatment of asthma. One of the benefits may be to reduce respiratory rate and hyperventilation. There does appear to be a small benefit in symptoms and bronchodilator use in controlled studies without improvement in lung function (Ducharme et al., 2004).

Homeopathy

There have been suggestions of improvement in some studies, either in symptoms without change in forced expiratory volume in 1 second (FEV1) or small changes in lung function, but no benefit in high-quality studies.

Ionisation

Inspiration of ionised air may have a small effect on lung function and may attenuate the response to exercise, but such effects are limited and the degree of ionisation is not achieved by the widely advertised home ionisers. There is even some suggestion that these may make nocturnal cough worse and there is no indication to use them.

Massage and spinal manipulation

These techniques have been popular but have not been shown to have any benefit in the few controlled studies.

Speleotherapy

Descent into subterranean environments is a common approach in Central and Eastern Europe. Some studies have shown short-term benefit but adequate controlled trials are needed. Moving to high altitudes where there is low pollution and allergen levels is a traditional approach with short-term benefits, but no evidence of a continued effect on return to the usual environment.

Traditional and herbal medicines

It is likely that some of these preparations contain potentially useful agents. However, there are difficulties in standardisation of products and some have been found to contain agents such as corticosteroids with the usual side effects.

References

Ducharme F, Schwartz Z, Hicks G, Kakuma R. Addition of anti-leukotriene agents to inhaled corticosteroids for chronic asthma. *Cochrane Database System Review* 2004; 2: CD003133.

Holt S, Suder A, Weatherall M, Cheng S, Shirtcliffe P, Beasley R. Dose-response of inhaled fluticasone propionate in adolescents and adults with asthma: meta-analysis. *British Medical Journal* 2001; 323: 253–256.

Leach CL. Improved delivery of inhaled steroids to the large and small airways. *Respiratory Medicine* 1998; 92 (Suppl A): 3–8.

O'Byrne PM, Bisgaard H, Godard PP *et al.* Budesonide/formoterol combination therapy as both maintenance and reliever medication in asthma. *American Journal of Respiratory and Critical Care Medicine* 2005; 171: 129–136.

Pauwels RA, Lofdahl CG, Postma DS *et al.* Effect of inhaled formoterol and budesonide on exacerbations of asthma. Eformoterol and Corticosteroids Establishing Therapy (FACET) International Study Group. *The New England Journal of Medicine* 1997; 337: 1405–1411.

Further reading

Adcock IM, Caraman G, Chung KF. New targets for drug development in asthma. *Lancet* 2008; 372: 1073–1087.

Cooper S, Oborne J, Newton S *et al.* Effect of two breathing exercises (Buteyko and pranayama) in asthma: a randomised controlled trial. *Thorax* 2003; 58: 674–679.

Ilowite J, Webb R, Friedman B *et al.* Addition of montelukast or salmeterol to fluticasone for protection against asthma attacks: a randomized, double-blind, multicenter study. *Annals of Allergy, Asthma & Immunology* 2004; 92: 641–648.

O'Byrne PM, Naya IP, Kallen A, Postma DS, Barnes PJ. Increasing doses of inhaled corticosteroids compared to adding long-acting inhaled beta2 agonists in achieving asthma control. *Chest* 2008; 134: 1192–1199.

Walker S, Monteil M, Phelan K, Lasserson TJ, Walters EH. Anti-IgE for chronic asthma in adults and children. *Cochrane Database System Review* 2006; Apr 19(2): CD003559.

CHAPTER 8

General Management of Acute Asthma

John Rees

Sherman Education Centre, Guy's Hospital, London, UK

OVERVIEW

- Some severe asthma attacks come on over minutes with no warning, but most develop over a period greater than 2 days
- Patients must be taught to seek help early rather than late in an acute exacerbation
- All asthmatic patients should be aware of what to do if they fail to get relief from their usual treatment
- An assessment of severity should be made using standard criteria
- A normal or high $PaCO_2$ is usually a sign of life-threatening asthma

---

Assessment of severity

The speed of onset of acute attacks varies. Some severe episodes come on over a period of minutes with no warning, although more often there is a background of deterioration over days or weeks. Eighty percent of episodes develop over a period greater than 2 days (Figure 8.1). This period during which control of the asthma deteriorates tends to be longer in older patients. A good early guide to developing problems is the need to use bronchodilator inhalers more often than usual or finding that they are less effective.

Peak flow monitoring

Deterioration in control can also be detected by measurement of peak flow at home; a drop in the peak flow or an increase in the diurnal variation of peak flow provides evidence of instability. Detecting these changes allows a change of treatment while the decline is slow and occurs before severe problems arise. Even if patients do not use their peak flow meter regularly it can be useful to confirm changes in symptoms. All asthmatic patients should be aware of what to do if they fail to get relief from their usual treatment. A written action plan should be available for patients and relatives, which should include trigger levels of peak flow as percentage of their best known or symptoms that require changes in treatment or consultation for further advice.

ABC of Asthma, 6th edition. By J. Rees, D. Kanabar and S. Pattani.
Published 2010 by Blackwell Publishing.

Breathlessness

The most common symptom is breathlessness, and there is more likely to be a sensation of difficulty in inspiration than in expiration. Some patients have a poor appreciation of changes in the degree of their airflow obstruction and will complain of few symptoms until they have developed moderately severe asthma. They are more likely to develop severe asthma and are at particular risk during acute attacks. When such patients are detected, they should be encouraged to use a peak flow meter regularly to provide objective evidence of their asthma control. This is a group in which regular peak flow monitoring is particularly important. Some studies of patients who have had life-threatening asthma show that patients with psychosocial problems, poor adherence to therapy and high levels of denial are over-represented compared with control asthmatics (Box 8.1).

Box 8.1 **Risk factors for severe acute asthma**

- Previous severe attacks
- Asthma severity (judged by medication needed)
- 'Brittle asthma'
- Poor compliance
- Psychiatric illness
- Denial of illness
- Obesity
- Psychosocial problems

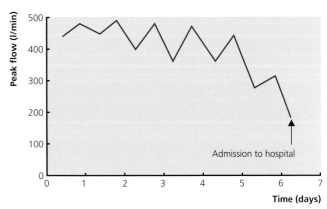

Figure 8.1 Gradual deterioration in peak flow in acute exacerbation.

As the severity of the asthma increases, breathlessness begins to interfere with simple functions. Exercise is limited and, later, eating and drinking are difficult. In severe attacks it will be difficult for the patient to speak in full sentences without gasping for breath between words. A knowledge of the pattern of previous attacks is important as the progress is often broadly similar in subsequent episodes.

Seeking help

Patients must be taught to seek help early rather than late in an acute exacerbation; it is easier to step in and prevent deterioration into severe asthma than to treat a full-blown attack. Patients and their families should be confident about the management of exacerbations – not only their immediate treatment but seeking further help and hospital admission. These should all be discussed before the first acute attack of asthma and be set out in a written asthma management plan (Box 8.2).

Box 8.2 **Responding to problems**

All patients with asthma should be aware of what to do if they fail to get relief from their usual treatment. Patients and relatives should have a written action plan that should include trigger levels of peak flow as percentage of their best known or symptoms that require changes in treatment or consultation for further advice.

Examination

Inability to speak will be obvious when taking the history. Respiratory rate is a useful sign and should be counted accurately; a rate of 25 beats per minute or above is a sign of severity (Boxes 8.3 and 8.4). Hypoxia severe enough to cause confusion occurs only in severe asthma and means that admission to hospital and supplemental oxygen are needed urgently. The pulse rate is also a useful guide to severity: tachycardia over 110 beats per minute is found in severe episodes although this sign may be less reliable in the elderly when pulse rates tend to remain low. In very severe attacks bradycardia may occur.

Box 8.3 **Initial assessment in acute asthma in adults**

Symptoms
Signs
- Breathlessness
- Cyanosis
- Respiratory rate
- Heart rate
- Blood pressure
- Chest examination
Respiratory function
- Peak expiratory flow (PEF) or FEV$_1$
- Comparison with patient's best or predicted
Oximetry
Blood gases (if saturation <93% or there are life-threatening features)

Chest X-ray if the following are present:
- Localising signs on examination
- Suspected pneumothorax
- Features suggesting pneumonia
- Failure to respond
- Ventilation required
Blood tests
- Full blood count
- Electrolytes
- Renal function

Box 8.4 **Assessment of severity in asthma**

Always err on the side of caution in the assessment. In general, those with acute severe asthma or life-threatening asthma should be referred to hospital. Other factors such as response to treatment, social circumstances or other medical conditions may influence decisions about place of treatment. Outside the hospital, the following features can be used to assess severity:

Near fatal asthma is indicated by a raised PaCO$_2$.

Life-threatening asthma (any one of the following):

- PEF <33% best or predicted
- SaO$_2$ <92%
- PaO$_2$ <8.0 kPa
- Normal PaCO$_2$ (i.e. not low)
- Silent chest
- Cyanosis
- Feeble respiratory effort
- Bradycardia
- Dysrhythmia
- Hypotension
- Exhaustion
- Confusion
- Coma

Acute severe asthma (any one of the following)

- PEF 33–50% best or predicted
- Respiratory rate ≥25/min
- Heart rate ≥110/min
- Inability to talk in sentences without breaths

Moderate exacerbation

- PEF 50–75% best or predicted
- No features of acute severe asthma

Pulsus paradoxus (a drop in systolic pressure of more than 10 mm Hg on inspiration) is a traditional measurement in acute asthma but is not useful in practice. Any evidence of circulatory embarrassment, such as hypotension, is an indication for admission to hospital.

Chest sounds

Examination of the chest itself shows a fast respiratory rate, over-inflation and wheezing. In very severe acute asthma, airflow may be too little for an audible wheeze, so a quiet chest during an acute attack is worrying rather than reassuring. It may also indicate a pneumothorax (although these are not common in acute asthma, they are difficult to diagnose clinically; a chest X-ray film must be taken if there is any doubt).

Peak flow readings

In severe attacks the peak flow rate may be unrecordable. Peak flow or forced expiratory volume (FEV) should be monitored throughout the attack and during recovery as they are reliable, simple guides to the effectiveness of treatment. Peak flow values are easier to interpret if the patient's usual or best readings are known.

Blood gases

An initial measurement of blood gases should be done in patients with asthma severe enough to warrant admission to hospital

(Box 8.5). Great care should be taken in obtaining arterial blood because some asthmatic patients who have had bad experiences of arterial puncture may delay attendance at hospital because of the memories of pain. In patients with mild attacks, a pulse oximeter should be used in the accident and emergency department. If saturation is 93% or above while breathing air and the patient does not have signs of severe asthma, then blood gas measurement can be omitted. In more severe cases, oxygen saturation by pulse oximeter can be used to assess progress after the first arterial gas measurement, provided the initial carbon dioxide tension was not raised and there is no sign of appreciable deterioration.

> **Box 8.5 Arterial blood gases in acute asthma**
>
> In hospital, blood gases provide extra information and PaO_2 <8 kPa or a normal $PaCO_2$ of 4.6–6.0 kPa (i.e. not the low $PaCO_2$ expected in milder attacks) are also features of life-threatening asthma.

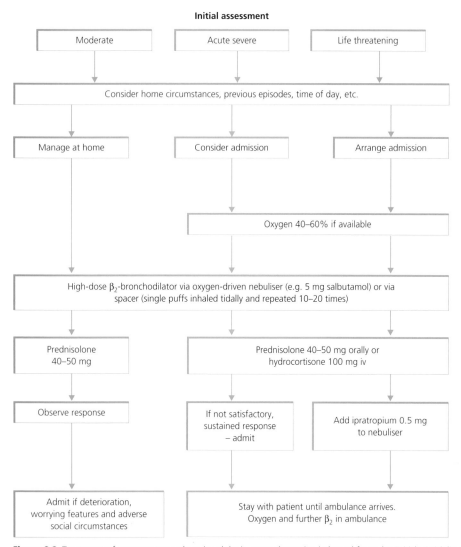

Figure 8.2 Treatment of acute severe asthma in adults in general practice (adapted from the British Guideline on the Management of Asthma. *Thorax* 2008; 63 (Suppl IV)).

Hypoxia and hypercapnia

Some hypoxia is usual and responds to supplemental oxygen. An arterial oxygen tension of less than 8 kPa on air is a mark of severity. As long as the patient does not have chronic obstructive pulmonary disease (COPD), there is no need to limit the concentration of supplemental oxygen. The arterial carbon dioxide tension is usually low in acute asthma; occasionally, particularly in children, it is high on admission, but quickly responds to treatment with a bronchodilator. However, hypercapnia is an alarming feature of acute asthma and failure either to reduce carbon dioxide retention during the first hour or to prevent its development during treatment is an indication that mechanical ventilation must be considered. The final decision on this depends on the overall clinical state of the patient rather than on the blood gas measurement alone.

Where to treat acute asthma

An acute attack of asthma is frightening; transfer to hospital might exacerbate symptoms by producing anxiety, and reassurance that treatment is available to relieve the attack is an important part of the management. It is not possible to lay down strict criteria for admission to hospital. The features of severity discussed above should, however, be assessed.

Most of the dangers of acute asthma come from a failure to appreciate the severity of an attack and the absence of suitable supervision and treatment to follow-up the initial response. Immediate improvement after the first nebuliser treatment may provide false reassurance, being followed quickly by the return of severe asthma, so continued observation is essential.

Initial treatment

It may be obvious on first seeing the patient that supplemental oxygen and hospital treatment are necessary (Figure 8.2). Treatment should be started while this is arranged. In less severe attacks, initial treatment should be given and, if the response is inadequate, hospital admission should be arranged. If the initial response is adequate, it may be possible to manage the patient at home if supervision is available. The primary treatment should then be followed up, usually by adequate bronchodilation and corticosteroids, and the response should be assessed by measurements of peak flow. Threshold for admission should be lowered if there has been a recent admission, previous severe attacks, poor patient perception of severity or poor social support.

Dangers of under-treatment

Most deaths from asthma occur when the patient or doctor has failed to appreciate the severity of the attack. When there is any doubt, it is safer to opt for vigorous treatment and admission to hospital. When treatment is given at home, the patient's condition must be assessed regularly and often until the exacerbation has settled. The reason for the acute exacerbation and the patient's response must always be reviewed.

Further reading

British Thoracic Society and the Scottish Intercollegiate Guidelines Network. British guideline on the management of asthma http://www.brit-thoracic.org.uk/docs/asthmafull.pdf.

CHAPTER 9

Treatment of Acute Asthma

John Rees

Sherman Education Centre, Guy's Hospital, London, UK

OVERVIEW

- Most problems in acute severe asthma result from under-treatment and failure to appreciate severity

- Forty to sixty percent oxygen should be given with a reservoir mask to achieve oxygen saturations above 94%

- A spacer device can deliver bronchodilators as effectively as a nebuliser in most cases of acute asthma

- Corticosteroids should be used early in acute attacks of asthma

- Discharge too early after an acute attack is associated with increased readmission and mortality

---

Introduction

The initial assessment of a patient with increased symptoms of asthma is very important. Most problems result from under-treatment and failure to appreciate severity. Monitor the peak flow rate and other signs before and after the first nebuliser treatment and then as appropriate (Figure 9.1). In hospital, peak flow should be monitored at least four times daily for the duration of the stay. A flow chart for the management of asthma at home is shown in Chapter 8 and a flow chart for management in hospital is shown later in this chapter. The various aspects of treatment are considered individually in this chapter.

Oxygen

Acute severe asthma is always associated with hypoxia, although cyanosis develops late and is a grave sign. Death in asthma is caused by severe hypoxia; oxygen should be given as soon as possible. It is very unusual to provoke carbon dioxide retention with oxygen treatment in asthma, so oxygen should be given freely aiming for saturations above 93% during transfer to hospital where blood gas measurement can be made. Masks can provide 40–60% oxygen.

Nebulisers should be driven by oxygen whenever possible. In older subjects with an exacerbation of chronic obstructive pulmonary disease (COPD) there is a potential danger of carbon dioxide retention. In these cases, treatment should begin with 24%

or 28% oxygen by Venturi mask until the results of blood gas measurements are available.

Details of oxygen delivery and target saturation should be written clearly on the prescription sheet. Nasal cannulae, simple facemasks or reservoir masks should be prescribed to obtain a target saturation of 94–98%

β-agonists

Adrenaline has been used in the treatment of asthma since just after the First World War. The specific short-acting β_2-agonists such as salbutamol and terbutaline have replaced the earlier non-selective preparations for acute use. There are no great differences in practice between the commonly used agents. If long-acting bronchodilators are used they can be continued during the attack.

Use and availability of nebulisers

In acute asthma, metered dose inhalers often lose their effectiveness. This is largely due to difficulties in the delivery of the drugs to the airways because of coordination problems and narrowing and occlusion of the airways.

An alternative method of giving β-agonist is necessary – usually by nebuliser or intravenously. A spacer device (e.g. Aerochamber,

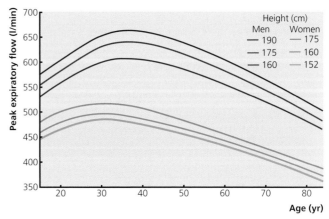

Figure 9.1 Predicted values for peak expiratory flow (adapted from Nunn AJ, Gregg I. *British Medical Journal* 1989; 298: 1068–1070).

ABC of Asthma, 6th edition. By J. Rees, D. Kanabar and S. Pattani. Published 2010 by Blackwell Publishing.

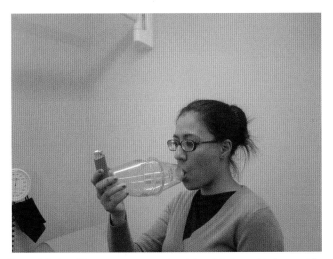

Figure 9.2 Attaching a spacer to a metered dose inhaler avoids the need for coordination between firing and inhalation.

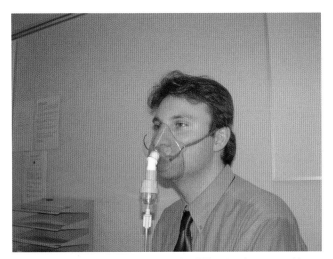

Figure 9.3 In acute asthma β-stimulants should be given by oxygen-driven nebuliser.

Nebuhaler or Volumatic) can be as effective as a nebuliser in most cases (Figure 9.2). Like the nebuliser, it has the advantage of removing the need to coordinate inhaler actuation and breathing. There is little or no difference in the effectiveness of drugs that are nebulised or given intravenously in acute severe asthma, so nebulisation is generally preferable.

It is helpful for general practitioners (GPs) to have nebulisers available for acute asthmatic attacks (Figure 9.3). β₂-agonists are best given by nebulisers driven by oxygen in acute asthma, as they may even worsen hypoxia slightly through an effect on the pulmonary vasculature. In general practice the use of oxygen as the driving gas is not usually practical. Domiciliary oxygen sets do not produce a flow rate adequate to drive most nebulisers. If available they can be used with nasal cannulae at the same time as an air driven nebuliser for a patient having an acute attack. Many ambulance services are able to give nebulised drugs and oxygen during transfer to hospital.

In hospital, nebulisers used to treat asthmatic patients should be driven by oxygen unless the patient has COPD with carbon dioxide

retention. The driving gas, flow rate, drug diluent and volume of fill should be clearly written on the prescription chart. Dilutions should always be done with saline to avoid bronchoconstriction from nebulisation of hypotonic solutions. There is no real advantage of nebulisation with a machine capable of producing intermittent positive pressure.

For adults the initial dose should be 5 mg salbutamol or its equivalent. This should be halved if the patient has ischaemic heart disease. It is essential to continue the intensive treatment after the first response; many of the problems in acute asthma arise because of complacency after the initial response to the first treatment. In severe attacks, the nebulisation may need to be repeated every 15 to 30 minutes and can be given continuously at 5–10 mg per hour with the same effect.

Parenteral delivery

If nebulised drugs are not effective then parenteral treatment should be considered. A reasonable plan is to give a β₂-agonist the first time, combine with an anticholinergic drug for the second nebulisation or initially in life-threatening asthma and move to intravenous bronchodilators if there is no improvement. If life-threatening features such as a raised carbon dioxide tension, an arterial oxygen tension less than 8 kPa on oxygen or a low pH are present, the intravenous agent should be considered from the start.

The bronchodilator given parenterally in an acute attack can be β₂-agonist or aminophylline; there is little to choose between them. If the patient has been on theophylline and a level is not immediately available it is safer to use the β₂-agonist. Salbutamol or terbutaline can be given intravenously over 10 minutes, or as an infusion, usually at 5 to 15 μg per minute. The adverse effects of tachycardia and tremor are much more common after intravenous injection than after nebulisation.

Anticholinergic agents

Ipratropium bromide is the only anticholinergic agent available in nebulised form in the United Kingdom (Figure 9.4). Nebulised ipratropium seems to be as effective as a nebulised β-agonist in acute asthma. The dose of ipratropium is 500 mcg and there are no problems with increased viscosity of secretions or mucociliary clearance at such doses. Ipratropium starts working more slowly than salbutamol; the peak response may not occur for 30 to 60 minutes.

Adverse reactions such as paradoxical bronchoconstriction have been reported occasionally. These were related mainly to the osmolality of the solution or to the preservatives and they have been corrected in the current preparations.

Although the combination of β-stimulant and anticholinergic agents produces a greater effect than use of a single agent, the difference is small and β₂-agonists are sufficient for most patients. It is reasonable to start with a β₂-agonist alone in moderate exacerbations and add ipratropium if the response to the first nebulisation is not considered adequate. If the initial assessment indicates that it is a severe or life-threatening attack then the combination should be used from the start. After stabilisation the ipratropium can be stopped.

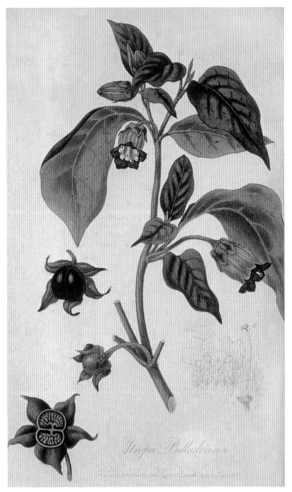

Figure 9.4 *Atropa belladonna* (deadly nightshade) contains several anticholinergic substances.

Table 9.1 Drug interactions with theophylline.

Drug	Effect
Increase in theophylline concentration	
Alcohol	Decreases theophylline clearance
Allopurinol	Decreased clearance
Cimetidine	Inhibits cytochrome P450, reducing clearance
Ciprofloxacin	As cimetidine
Interferon alfa	Marked decrease in clearance
Macrolides (erythromycin)	Decreased clearance
Oestrogen	Decreased clearance
Ticlopidine	Decreased clearance, concentrations may rise by 60%
Zafirlukast	Decreased clearance
Decrease in theophylline concentration	
Carbamazepine	50% increase in clearance
Cigarette smoking	Increased clearance around 30%
Phenytoin	Up to 70% increased clearance
Rifampicin	Increases cytochrome P450, increasing theophylline clearance up to 80%
Effect on other drugs	
Benzodiazepines	Larger doses of benzodiazepine may be required, effects may increase if theophylline is discontinued
Lithium	Lithium clearance increased
Pancuronium	Antagonised by theophylline, larger doses may be necessary

Methylxanthines

Aminophylline is an effective bronchodilator in acute asthma but most studies have shown that it is no more effective than a β_2-agonist given by mobilisation or intravenously. There are more problems with its use than with nebulised drugs and it should be reserved for patients with life-threatening features or who have failed to respond to nebulised drugs. Toxic effects are common and can occur with drug concentrations in or just above the therapeutic range. Concentrations are difficult to predict from the dose given because of individual differences in metabolic rate and interactions with drugs such as nicotine, cimetidine, erythromycin and ciprofloxacin (Table 9.1).

The position is further complicated if patients are already taking oral theophyllines. The usual starting dose for intravenous aminophylline is 5 mg/kg given over 20 to 30 minutes. If the patient has taken oral theophylline or aminophylline in the previous 24 hours and a blood concentration is not available then the initial dose should be omitted or halved. A continuous infusion is then given at a rate of 0.5–0.7 mg/kg/hr though this dose should be reduced if the patient also has kidney or liver disease. If intravenous treatment is necessary for more than 24 hours then

blood concentrations should be measured and the rate adjusted as necessary.

Corticosteroids

Corticosteroids are effective in preventing the development of acute asthma.

Oral delivery

Oral prednisolone should be given if control of asthma is deteriorating despite usual regular treatment (Box 9.1). A single oral dose of prednisolone, 40 to 50 mg according to body weight, should be given each day for at least 5 days until recovery according to the speed of the response. If this opportunity is missed and an acute attack of asthma does develop, corticosteroids are still an important element in treatment. Fatal attacks of asthma are associated with failure to prescribe any or adequate doses of corticosteroids. No noticeable response occurs for 4 to 6 hours, so corticosteroids should be started as early as possible and intensive bronchodilator treatment used while waiting for them to take effect.

> **Box 9.1 Adverse effects of short course of oral corticosteroids**
>
> - Fluid retention
> - Hyperglycaemia
> - Indigestion
> - Sleep disturbance
> - Steroid-induced psychosis
> - Susceptibility to severe herpes zoster
> - Weight gain

Intravenous delivery

In most cases oral corticosteroids are adequate, but when there are life-threatening features or difficulties with swallowing or absorption intravenous hydrocortisone should be used in an initial dose of 100 mg followed by 100 mg six hourly for 24 hours. Prednisolone should be started at a dose of 40 to 50 mg daily whether or not hydrocortisone is used (50 mg prednisolone is equivalent to 200 mg hydrocortisone). If the patient is first seen at home and transferred to hospital, the first dose of corticosteroid should be given together with initial bronchodilator treatment before leaving home.

Length of steroid course

When intensive initial treatment has been required prednisolone should be maintained at a dose of 40 mg per day for at least 5 days. One to three weeks of treatment may be needed to obtain the maximal response with deflation to normal lung volumes and loss of excessive diurnal variations of peak flow. There are few side effects of such short courses of corticosteroids. Increased appetite, fluid retention, gastrointestinal upset and psychological disturbance are the most common. Exposure to herpes zoster may produce severe infections in susceptible individuals. Steroids can be stopped abruptly after courses lasting up to 3 weeks. Tapering off the dose is not needed for adrenal suppression or does not help prevent relapse although many patients are used to such regimes. Inhaled steroids should be continued or started during inpatient treatment in accordance with the plans for routine management.

Magnesium

Intravenous magnesium sulphate has been shown to be effective and safe in acute asthma. Magnesium sulphate is given as an infusion, at a dose of 1.2–2 g over 20 minutes. It provides a possible additional therapy in acute severe asthma in hospital when the initial response to nebulised bronchodilators is inadequate or when the initial assessment indicates life-threatening or near fatal asthma. Doses can be repeated for episodes of deterioration in hospital.

Fluid and electrolytes

Patients with acute asthma tend to be dehydrated because they are often too breathless to drink and because fluid loss from the respiratory tract is increased. Dehydration increases the viscosity of mucus, making plugging of the airways more likely, so intravenous fluid replacement is often necessary. Three litres should be given during the first 24 hours if little oral fluid is being taken.

Potassium supplements

Increased alveolar ventilation, sympathomimetic drugs and corticosteroids all tend to lower the serum potassium concentration. This is the most common disturbance of electrolytes in acute asthma; the serum potassium concentration should be monitored and supplements given as necessary.

Antibiotics

Upper respiratory tract infections are the most common trigger factors for acute asthma and most of these are viral. In only a few cases are exacerbations of asthma precipitated by bacterial infection.

There is no evidence of benefit from the routine use of antibiotics. They should be reserved for patients in whom there is presumptive evidence of infection – such as fever, neutrophils in the blood or sputum or radiological changes, although all these features may occur in acute attacks without bacterial infection.

Controlled ventilation

Patients with acute severe asthma who need hospital admission should be treated in an area equipped to deal with acute medical emergencies, with adequate nursing and medical supervision. If hypoxia is worsening, hypercapnia is present or patients are exhausted or drowsy, then they should be nursed in an intensive care unit.

Occasionally, mechanical ventilation may be necessary for a short time while the treatment takes effect. It is usually needed because the patient becomes exhausted; experience and careful observation are necessary to judge the right time to begin ventilatory support. Non-invasive ventilation may be tried in expert hands in an intensive care unit.

High inflation pressures and long expiratory times may make ventilation difficult in asthmatic patients, but most experienced units have good results, provided that the decision to ventilate the patient is made electively and is not precipitated by respiratory arrest. When patients being mechanically ventilated fail to improve on adequate treatment, bronchial lavage may occasionally be considered to reopen airways that have become plugged by mucus. In very severe unresponsive cases other treatments such as inhalational anaesthetics may be helpful, or a mixture of helium and oxygen may improve airflow while the other treatment takes effect.

Other factors

Most patients with acute severe asthma improve with these measures (Figure 9.5). Occasionally physiotherapy may be useful to help patients cough up thick plugs of sputum, but mucolytic agents to change the nature of the secretions do not help.

An episode of asthma is frightening. The dangerous use of sedatives such as morphine was common before effective treatment became available. Unfortunately, this practice still continues, with occasional fatal consequences. Treatment of agitation should be aimed at reversing the asthma precipitating it, not at producing respiratory depression.

Discharge from hospital

Discharge too early is associated with increased readmission and with mortality. Patients should have stopped nebuliser treatment and be using their own inhalers, with the proper technique checked, for at least 24 hours before discharge (Box 9.2). Ideally, peak flow should be above 75% of the patient's predicted or best-known

Immediate management
Oxygen 40–60%
Salbutamol 5 mg or terbutaline and
  ipratropium 0.5 mg by oxygen driven
  nebuliser
Prednisolone 40–50 mg orally or
  hydrocortisone 100 mg intravenously
No sedation
Consider need for chest radiograp

Life–threatening features
• Peak flow <33% Predicted or best
• Silent chest, feeble respiratory effort
• Cyanosis, SaO$_2$ <92%
• Bradycardia, hypotension, dysrhythmia
• Exhausion, confusion, coma
• PCO$_2$ ≥ 4.6 kPa, PO$_2$ ≤ 8 kPa, acidosis

If life–threatening features are present
• Discuss with ICU team
• IV magnesium sulphate 1.2–2 g iv
  over 20 min
• Frequent or continuous β$_2$-agoinst
  nebulisation

Improving
Continue
• Oxygen
• Prednisolone 40–50 mg daily
• β-agonist and ipratropium 4–6 hourly

Not improving after 15–30 min
Continue
Oxygen and steroids
β-agonist up to every 15 min or
  continuously
Ipratropium bromide 0.5 mg 4–6 hourly

Monitor
• Peak flow before and after nebulisations
• Oximetry (keep saturation >92%)
• Blood gas tensions if initial PaO$_2$
  <8 kPa and saturation <93%
  or PaCO2 normal or high
  or patient deteriorates

If still not improving
Aminophylline infusion 0.5 mg/kg/hr
(monitor concentrations if longer than
24 hr)
or
salbutamol or terbutaline infusion 5 to
15 µg/min
Discuss with ICU team

Figure 9.5 Treatment of acute severe asthma in hospital (adapted from guidelines from the British Thoracic Society and Scottish Intercollegiate Guidelines Network).

reading. Diurnal variability should be below 25%. A few patients may never lose their morning dips and may have to be discharged with them still present (Figure 9.6).

Box 9.2 **Discharge after acute severe asthma admission**

Patients discharged should have the following:

• Planned discharge medication for 24 hours before discharge
• Inhaler technique checked
• Peak expiratory flow (PEF) >75% best or predicted
• PEF diurnal variation <25%
• Oral and inhaled steroids
• Bronchodilators
• PEF meter
• Written asthma management plan
• Discharge summary for GP
• GP follow-up within 2 working days
• Chest clinic follow-up within 4 weeks
• Circumstances of acute exacerbation and patient response explored

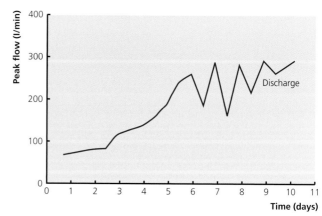

Figure 9.6 Peak flow during recovery from acute attack.

For every patient the reason for the acute episode should be sought and appropriate changes made in their routine treatment and in their response to any deterioration in an attempt to avoid similar attacks in the future. Patients with an acute attack of asthma should be looked after or at least seen by a physician with an interest in respiratory disease during their inpatient stay. Follow-up should be arranged and a respiratory specialist nurse will be helpful in education, management and support.

Subsequent management

At the time of their discharge, patients should be stable on the treatment that they will take at home. They should leave with a plan of further management. This should include advice on asthma, symptoms and peak flow measurement and a plan to respond to deterioration in the control of their asthma. The GP should be informed of the admission and the subsequent plans and should see the patient within two working days.

Hospital follow-up

The patient should return to the chest clinic within a month. Good communication between hospital and the GP is vital around this vulnerable period – telephone, fax and electronic links may help.

Further reading

British Thoracic Society. Emergency Oxygen Guideline Group Guideline for emergency oxygen use in adult patients. *Thorax* 2008; 63 (Suppl VI).

Silverman RA, Osborn H, Runge J *et al.*; Acute Asthma/Magnesium Study Group. IV magnesium sulfate in the treatment of acute severe asthma: a multicenter randomized controlled trial. *Chest* 2002; 122: 489–497.

CHAPTER 10

Methods of Delivering Drugs

John Rees

Sherman Education Centre, Guy's Hospital, London, UK

OVERVIEW

- With the combinations of drug and inhaler available it is possible for nearly all patients to take drugs by inhalation
- Even when a metered dose inhaler (MDI) is used properly, only about 10% of the drug reaches the airways below the larynx
- Inhaler technique should be checked regularly since errors can develop and interfere with treatment
- Chlorofluorocarbon (CFC)-free beclometasone MDIs need to be prescribed by brand because of differences in lung deposition
- Spacer devices help coordination problems with MDIs and reduce pharyngeal deposition

Various inhaler devices and formulations have been developed to deliver drugs efficiently, minimise side effects and simplify use. With over 100 combinations of drug and inhaler available, it is possible for nearly all patients to take drugs by inhalation, but there is scope for confusion for patients and prescribers. All the available devices used appropriately can provide adequate drug to the airways, but inhalers should only be prescribed with confidence that the patient can use the device satisfactorily. This should be rechecked on subsequent visits since errors can develop and interfere with treatment. Even after training, at least one-third of patients continue to make errors in their inhalation technique in most studies. The scores used in assessing technique may not all relate similarly to clinical effectiveness, but some result in no drug delivery and poor technique is related to poor asthma control. Some drugs such as leukotriene receptor antagonists and theophylline cannot be given by inhalation.

Metered dose inhalers

Inhalers deliver the drug directly to the airways. Even when an MDI is used properly only about 10% of the drug reaches the airways below the larynx (Figures 10.1 and 10.2). Nearly all the rest of the drug gets no further than the oropharynx and is swallowed. This swallowed portion may be absorbed from the gastrointestinal tract but drugs such as inhaled corticosteroids are largely removed by

first-pass metabolism in the liver. Absorption directly from the lung bypasses liver metabolism.

An MDI should be shaken and then fired into the mouth shortly after the start of a slow full inspiration. At full inflation the breath should be held for 10 seconds. The technique should be checked periodically. At least a quarter of patients have difficulty using an MDI and the problems increase with

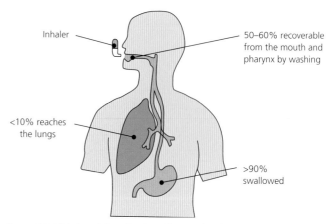

Inhaler

50–60% recoverable from the mouth and pharynx by washing

<10% reaches the lungs

>90% swallowed

Figure 10.1 Inhalers deliver the drug direct to the airways.

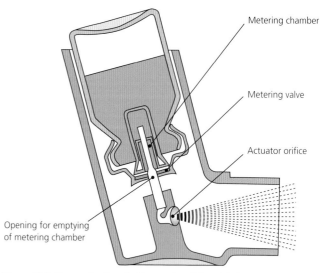

Metering chamber

Metering valve

Actuator orifice

Opening for emptying of metering chamber

Figure 10.2 The mechanisms inside a metered dose inhaler.

ABC of Asthma, 6th edition. By J. Rees, D. Kanabar and S. Pattani.
Published 2010 by Blackwell Publishing.

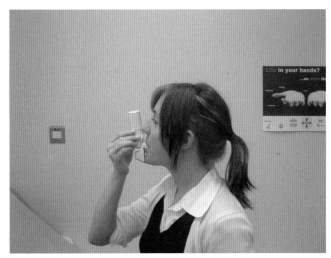

Figure 10.3 The autoinhaler is triggered by inspiratory airflow. Breath-actuated metered dose inhalers are available for β-agonists, anticholinergics, cromoglicate and corticosteroids.

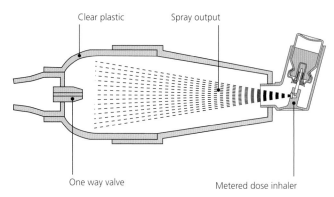

Figure 10.4 An extension tube (spacer) used with a metered dose inhaler. Some large volume spacers are being replaced by smaller volume devices.

age. The common problems are coordination of firing with inspiration. The 'cold Freon effect', stopping inspiration when the inhaler activates, is much less common with replacement of CFC-containing inhalers. Arthritic patients can find it hard to activate MDIs and may be helped by a Haleraid device, which responds to squeezing, or be given a breath-actuated or dry powder system.

Breath-actuated aerosol inhalers

Breath-actuated MDIs are available for most classes of drug (Figure 10.3). The pressurised canister is actuated via a spring triggered by inspiratory airflow. The devices respond to a low flow rate and are useful for those who have difficulty coordinating actuation and breathing. Errors are less frequent than with MDIs. They require a propellant similar to that caused in a standard inhaler.

Metered dose inhaler propellants

Most current MDIs have now moved from CFC propellants. The production, import and use of CFCs have been stopped in most developed countries because of the effect on the ozone layer. There is a temporary exemption for medical use under the Montreal Protocol, but CFC inhalers are being removed now that adequate non-CFC products are available.

The challenge has been to develop safe alternatives that are as convenient, effective and clinically equivalent. The process of development of alternative propellants was more of a problem than first appreciated, particularly for inhaled steroids. Adaptations to the method of adding the drug to the propellant and to the valve and jet mechanisms have been necessary. Hydrofluoroalkanes 134 and 227 are used in the new devices.

Short- and long-acting β-agonists, inhaled steroids and combinations are now available in HFA-containing MDIs. Each new device has to be tested carefully since total and regional delivery to the lung will differ with the new devices. The beclometasone product QVar is prescribed at half the dose of a conventional MDI because of its smaller particle size, resulting in better lung deposition. Other preparations are substituted in the ratio of 1:1. Patients will notice differences in the speed of the aerosol cloud and taste.

The switch to CFC-free MDIs should be taken as an opportunity to review patient understanding, inhaler technique and general asthma management.

Spacer devices

The coordination of firing and inspiration becomes slightly less important when a short extension tube is used. This may help if problems are minor but a larger reservoir removes the need for coordination of breathing and actuation (Figure 10.4). The inhaler is fixed into the chamber and breath is taken from a one-way valve at the other end of the chamber. Inhalation should be as soon as possible after each actuation, certainly within 30 seconds; tidal breathing is as effective as deep breaths. In young children they can be used with a facemask.

Pharyngeal deposition is greatly reduced as the faster particles strike the walls of the chamber, not the mouth. Evaporation of propellant from the larger and slower particles produces a small-sized aerosol that penetrates further out into the lungs and deposits a greater proportion of drug beyond the larynx. This reduces the risk of oral candidiasis and dysphonia with inhaled corticosteroids and reduces potential problems with systemic absorption from the gastrointestinal tract. Spacers should be used routinely when doses of inhaled steroid of more than 800 μg daily are given by MDI.

Most devices are cumbersome, but this is not a great disadvantage for twice daily treatment such as corticosteroids. Chambers can be used as effectively as nebulisers in mild to moderate exacerbations of asthma. Output characteristics of MDIs vary and inhalers and extension tubes need to be matched appropriately. It cannot be assumed that results transfer to different combinations.

Electrostatic charge can reduce drug delivery. Chambers should be washed in detergent and left to air dry rather than be wiped dry, just once a month and changed every 6–12 months. Metal chambers without static charge can also be used (Box 10.1).

Dry powder inhalers

Dry powder inhalers (DPIs) of various types are available for β-agonists, sodium cromoglicate, corticosteroids, anticholinergic agents and combinations (Figure 10.5). Because inspiratory airflow releases the fine powder, many problems of coordination are avoided and there are none of the environmental worries of MDIs. The dry powder makes some patients cough. The Turbohaler contains drug with no carrier and patients may feel that nothing is coming from the device. It has good lung deposition but requires a flow rate of >60 l/min, achieved easily by most patients.

The problems of reloading for each dose have been eased by the development of multiple dose units with up to 200 doses, and most DPIs have a dose counter that helps the patient to know when the inhaler needs renewing and provides a compliance monitor.

Soft mist inhalers

Soft mist inhalers (SMIs) contain liquid but no propellants and produce a slow-moving aerosol cloud (the soft mist). They are fired by the patient with inspiration but coordination is easier because of the slow velocity and the long duration.

Nebulisers

Nebulisers can be driven by compressed gas (jet nebuliser) or an ultrasonically vibrating crystal (ultrasonic nebuliser). They provide a way of giving inhaled drugs to those unable to use any other device – for example, the very young – or in acute attacks when inspiratory flow is limited.

Nebulisers also offer a convenient way of delivering a higher dose to the airways (Figure 10.6). Generally, about 12% of the drug leaving the chamber enters the lungs but most of the dose stays in the apparatus or is wasted in expiration. Delivery depends on the type of nebuliser chamber, the flow rate at which it is driven and the volume in the chamber. In most cases, flow rates of less than 6 l/min in a jet nebuliser give too large a particle and nebulise too slowly. Some chambers have a reservoir and valve system to reduce loss to the surrounding room during expiration.

In many situations, equivalent effects can be obtained with MDI and a spacer but patients often feel confidence in their nebuliser.

Tablets and syrups

Tablets and syrups are available for oral use. This route is necessary for theophyllines and leukotriene antagonists, which cannot be inhaled effectively. Very young children who are unable to inhale drugs can take the sugar-free liquid preparations. Slow-release tablets are used when a prolonged action is needed, particularly for nocturnal asthma in which theophyllines can be helpful. Various slow-release mechanisms or long-acting drugs have been developed to maintain even blood concentrations (Figure 10.7).

Bambuterol is a pro-drug of terbutaline which can be given once daily at night in those unable to use the inhaled route. Tablets avoid the need to learn the coordination needed for inhalers and might

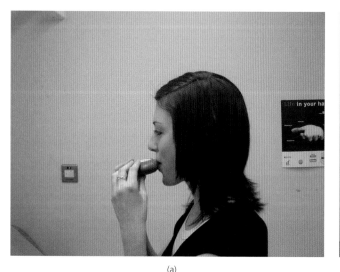

(a)

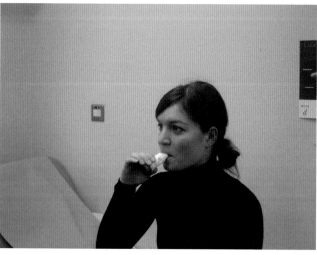

(b)

Figure 10.5 Dry powder inhalers are used for delivery of inhaled drugs. Two commonly used devices are the (a) accuhaler and the (b) turbohaler.

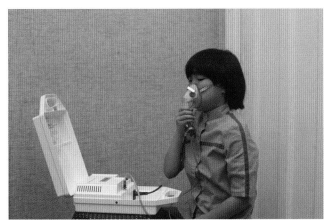

Figure 10.6 The use of nebulisers must be associated with careful instructions on use and hygiene as well as arrangements for maintenance and support.

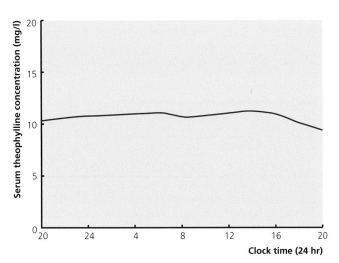

Figure 10.7 Steady theophylline concentrations in the therapeutic range can be obtained with 12-hourly slow-release preparations (reproduced with permission from Ferrari M *et al*. Effect of once daily and twice daily sustained release theophylline formulations on day-time variation of bronchial hyper-responsiveness in asthmatic patients. *Thorax* 1997: 52; 969–974).

allow delivery to lung tissue beyond blocked airways but at the expense of potential side effects from body distribution.

Injections and infusions

Injections are used for the treatment of acute attacks. Subcutaneous injections may be useful in emergencies when nebulisers are unavailable. Occasional patients with severe chronic asthma seem to benefit from the high levels of β-stimulant obtained with subcutaneous infusion through a portable pump (Figure 10.8). Rates

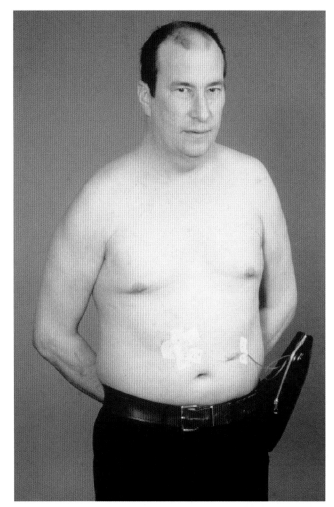

Figure 10.8 In severe cases β$_2$-agonists can be delivered by subcutaneous infusion.

may need to be adjusted, depending on severity. The infusion site is changed by the patient every 1 to 3 days.

Further reading

D'Alonzo GE, Smolensky MH, Feldman S *et al*. Twenty-four hour lung function in adult patients with asthma. Chronoptimized theophylline therapy once-daily dosing in the evening versus conventional twice-daily dosing. *The American Review of Respiratory Disease* 1990; 142: 84–90.

Giraud V, Roche N. Misuse of corticosteroid metered-dose inhalers is associated with decreased asthma stability. *European Respiratory Journal* 2002; 19: 246–251.

Pitcairn G, Reader S, Pavia D, Newman S. Deposition of corticosteroid aerosol in the human lung by Respimat Soft Mist inhaler compared to deposition by metered dose inhaler or by Turbohaler dry powder inhaler. *Journal of Aerosol Medicine* 2005; 18: 264–272.

Virchow JC, Crompton GK, Dal Negro R *et al*. Importance of inhaler devices in the management of airway disease. *Respiratory Medicine* 2008; 102: 10–19.

CHAPTER 11

Definition, Prevalence and Prevention

Dipak Kanabar

Evelina Children's Hospital, Guy's and St Thomas' Hospitals, London, UK

OVERVIEW

- Childhood asthma is most likely a spectrum of disorders
- A good clinical history is important in diagnosing childhood asthma
- Asthma affects one in six children at some point in their lives
- Atopy is probably the single strongest risk factor for asthma – exposure to relevant allergens in infancy or childhood may predispose a person to continued allergic responses later
- The hygiene hypothesis is an attractive hypothesis to explain rising prevalence of childhood asthma

Defining asthma in children

Western Europe has seen a dramatic increase in children suffering from asthma. Not only has the prevalence increased but also the severity of the illness. It is likely that events in early life lead to changes in the lung and immune systems which predispose the child to chronic asthmatic symptoms. It is becoming increasingly apparent that asthma is a spectrum disorder and probably has many definitions, however a working definition is given in Box 11.1.

Box 11.1 ICS report

The International Consensus Report on the Diagnosis and Management of Asthma gives the following definition: 'Asthma is a chronic inflammatory disorder of the airway in which many cells play a role, in particular mast cells, eosinophils, and T lymphocytes. In susceptible individuals this inflammation causes recurrent episodes of wheezing, breathlessness, chest tightness, and cough particularly at night and or in the early morning. These symptoms are usually associated with widespread but variable airflow limitation that is at least partly reversible either spontaneously or with treatment. The inflammation also causes an associated increase in airway responsiveness to a variety of stimuli.'

Childhood asthma is most likely a spectrum of disorders characterised by episodes of cough, wheeze, shortness of breath and exercise-induced wheeze. Wheezy episodes in children are a common phenomenon and up to 30% of children under the age of 5 may wheeze at some time point.

Labelling a child as asthmatic can still cause anxiety within the family and controversy among paediatricians (Figure 11.1). Most children under 5 presenting with asthmatic symptoms (see International Consensus Report) are either transient early wheezers or non-atopic wheezers, without a family or personal history of

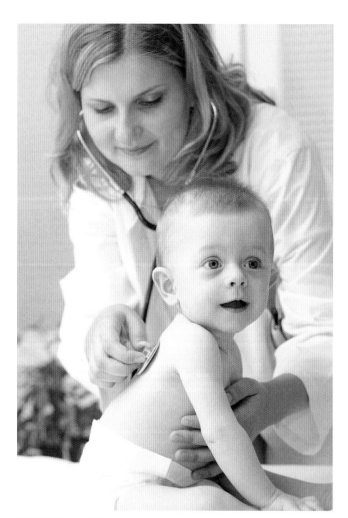

Figure 11.1 A definition of asthma.

ABC of Asthma, 6th edition. By J. Rees, D. Kanabar and S. Pattani.
Published 2010 by Blackwell Publishing.

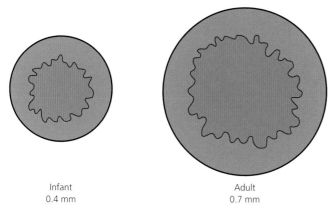

Infant
0.4 mm

Adult
0.7 mm

Figure 11.2 Comparative diameter of bronchioles.

atopy and tend to outgrow their wheezy symptoms at an early age (<7 years).

Atopic (immunoglobulin E (IgE)-associated) wheezers have raised IgE concentrations, positive radioallergosorbent (RAST) and skin prick tests and raised exhaled nitric oxide (FE_{NO}) concentrations.

Presenting symptoms

For example, respiratory syncitial virus (RSV) bronchiolitis itself causes wheezing and up to half of affected children will go on to develop recurrent episodic wheeze. Many children have mild wheezing during viral infections (virus-associated wheeze), but their prognosis is better than that of children who show bronchial hyper-reactivity to methacholine (non-atopic wheezers). In addition, the airways of preschool children are small relative to lung size (Figure 11.2). The airways and chest walls are also less rigid, so during expiration, they are more likely than those of older children to collapse, or become obstructed by desquamated airway epithelial cells and secretions or mucosal changes that are not the result of an inflammatory process like asthma.

Older children can describe symptoms of cough, wheeze, dyspnoea and chest tightness, and confirm whether there is an improvement with bronchodilator and steroid therapy. In addition, peak flow measurements, forced expiratory volume in 1 second (FEV1) by spirometry, exercise testing and recordings of diurnal variations will assist diagnosis.

Thus, in practice, in the absence of an easily recognised or readily available diagnostic marker, a clinical diagnosis of asthma usually relies on a combination of history of characteristic symptoms and evidence of airway lability and a reduction in symptoms after treatment with a short-acting β_2-agonist showing reversible airflow obstruction.

Prevalence of asthma

Asthma is the most common chronic disease of childhood. About one in six (17%) or more children aged between 2 and 15 years in the United Kingdom have symptoms of asthma at some time in their lives which requires treatment.

Is prevalence increasing or reaching a plateau?

While several epidemiological studies show that the prevalence of asthma and other atopic disorders such as eczema and hayfever is increasing in many countries throughout the world more recent studies indicate that, perhaps in the Western world at least, prevalence rates are reaching a plateau (Figure 11.3).

The observation that all forms of allergic disease have increased simultaneously suggests an increase in host susceptibility, rather than a rise in allergic sensitisation. Associations between the prevalence of asthma and small family size, environmental exposure to cigarette smoke, affluence, reduced cross infection and BCG status (decreased asthma with BCG vaccine) are all recognised and, coupled with our understanding of the immunology of asthma, hint at the possibility of factors either in utero or in early life, which might modify an individual's atopic tendency.

Based on self-reported data, international comparison studies (International Study of Asthma and Allergies in Childhood [ISAAC] phases I and III) have placed the United Kingdom near the top of the world league of asthma and allergy prevalence (Figure 11.4) and while there is some objective data to support large differences between the United Kingdom and countries such as Albania, it is not clear why other westernised nations with low levels of air pollution (e.g. New Zealand) also appear near the top of the table.

Phase III of ISACC confirms that English-speaking countries and Western Europe have recently seen a decrease in asthma prevalence, whereas regions where prevalence was previously low (Africa, Latin America and parts of Asia) have seen an increase (Figure 11.3).

Public health issues

In terms of burden of disease, childhood asthma presents a serious public health problem. More than half of all cases of asthma present before the age of 10, and over 30% of children experience a wheezing illness during the first few years of life. More absence from school is caused by asthma than any other chronic condition; 30% of asthmatic children miss more than 3 weeks of schooling each year. Asthma influences educational attainment even in children of above average intelligence, the extent of this adverse effect being related to severity of the disease.

Reasons for the increasing global prevalence

It is unlikely that there is a single cause and effect association to account for the rising global burden of asthma and atopic disorders. Recent immunological studies, however, have indicated that the first 3 years of life (including life before birth) are probably the most critical in terms of environmental influences on the development of the asthma phenotype. For example, there are strong links between cigarette smoking in pregnancy and narrow airways in the offspring, and the risk of a child developing asthma is more closely associated with allergy in the mother than in the father.

Further data from ISAAC phase III suggests that use of paracetamol in the first year of life and in later childhood, is associated with an increased risk of symptoms of asthma and other atopic disorders.

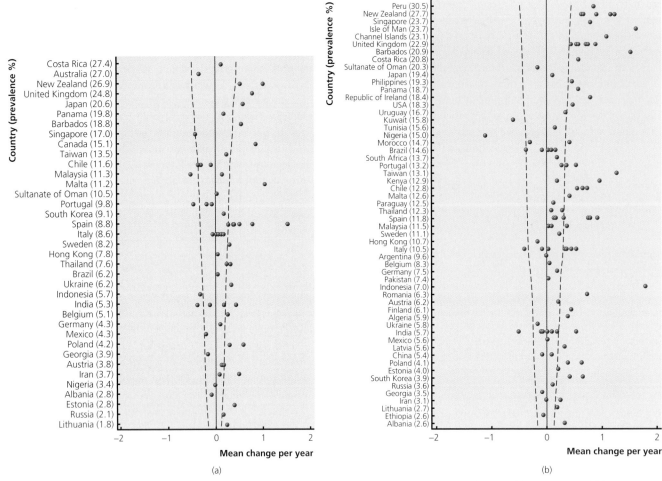

Figure 11.3 Ranking plot showing the change per year in the lifetime prevalence of asthma ('asthma ever') in children aged (a) 6–7 years and (b) 13–14 years for each centre by country, with countries ordered by their mean prevalence (for all centres combined) across phase I and phase III. The plot also shows the confidence interval about zero change for a given level of prevalence (i.e. the mean prevalence across phases I and III) given a sample size of 3000 and no cluster sampling effect. Reproduced with permission from Pearce N et al. Thorax 2007; 62: 758–766.

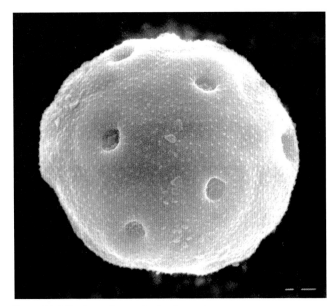

Figure 11.4 Electron micrograph of pollen grains.

Changes such as those in housing that allow proliferation of house dust mite, the effects of outdoor and indoor pollutants such as cigarette smoke, dietary changes, low birth weight and prematurity may all account for some of the increased prevalence. To account for the increase in disease prevalence from 10% to 15% (such as has occurred in the United Kingdom over the last 30 years), however, the proportion of the population exposed to these hazards would need to have increased from 10% to nearly 70%, suggesting that other, as yet unidentified, risk factors may be operating.

The relevance of atopy

Atopy, defined as the predisposition to raise specific IgE to common allergens (such as house dust mite, wheat and cat dander), is probably the single strongest risk factor for asthma, carrying up to a 20-fold increased risk of asthma in atopic individuals compared with non-atopic individuals. The strongest association is with maternal atopy – a maternal history of asthma or rhinitis, or both – and is a significant risk factor for late childhood onset asthma and recurrent wheezing (Figures 11.4 and 11.5).

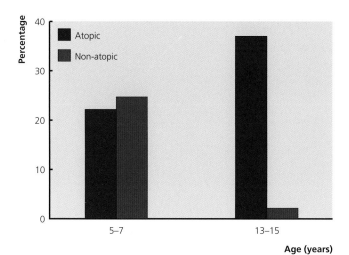

Figure 11.5 Atopy in children with bronchial hyper-reactivity.

A routine enquiry should be made about other atopic disorders such as atopic dermatitis (eczema), food allergies and rhinitis as they may be coexisting morbidities in a child with allergy-associated asthma.

Lymphocytes

T lymphocytes – in particular T-helper type 2 (Th2) lymphocytes – are also believed to be important in the pathogenesis of asthma. The fetal immune system is primarily polarised towards a Th2 response as a result of interleukin 4 and 10 (IL-4 and IL-10) production by the placenta. Furthermore, T lymphocytes isolated from cord blood of newborn babies of atopic mothers are able to respond to aeroallergens, suggesting that they may have been exposed to antigens ingested by the mother and transferred across the placenta in the last trimester of pregnancy.

During early childhood, environmental allergens – in particular intestinal microflora – are thought to influence the immune deviation of T-helper cells towards the Th1 type in non-atopic children and towards the Th2 type in atopic children. In atopic children with recurrent wheezing illness, bronchoalveolar lavage studies indicate increased mast cell and eosinophil concentrations in children as young as 3. Up to the age of 10, the peripheral blood mononuclear cell response to specific stimulation in children who develop atopic disease is deficient in its capacity to generate interferon gamma (IFNγ), thereby causing upregulation of Th2 responses and an allergic phenotype.

Early exposure to infections

Children growing up in rural and farming communities are much less likely to develop atopy and bronchial hyper-responsiveness than children raised in inner city areas. There is an inverse association between socio-economic status and asthma and allergy, and firstborn children have a higher prevalence of asthma than their siblings, with the assumption that children from higher social classes and firstborns are exposed to fewer infections in early life.

Observations such as these make the 'hygiene hypothesis' an attractive model when explaining the general rise in atopic disorders.

The 'hygiene hypothesis' argues that the increase in atopic asthma is due to a decrease in exposure to infection in early life. Frequent infections in childhood generate Th1 cytokines such as the interleukins IL-12, IL-18 and IFNγ, and these in turn inhibit the growth of Th2 cells, thus preventing development of the atopic asthma phenotype.

Prospects for prevention

Allergen avoidance studies such as the Isle of Wight study, where infants born to mothers with a strong family history of atopy were randomised to receive prophylaxis, with the mother eating a hypoallergenic diet and breastfeeding or giving a soya milk preparation to their babies, showed a significant decrease in the prevalence of eczema and a positive skin prick test to aeroallergen and dietary factors, but no sustained benefit in relation to reduction in asthma.

Other environmental avoidance studies have shown a reduction in respiratory symptoms in the first year of life, but subsequent results showed a paradoxical effect of increased allergy but better lung function.

Dietary manipulation (e.g. introduction of fish in the diet or fish oil supplementation) has shown some positive results in reducing the risk of eczema. Breastfeeding is still advised in all children not only for its other health benefits, but also for a preventative effect in development of asthma it may have in those children born to atopic families or in babies identified by high cord blood IgE, although the evidence is not conclusive (Figure 11.6).

These results seem to indicate that the development of asthma is a combination of genetic susceptibility and exposure in early life to allergic stimuli and pollutants that augment a Th2 immune response. Once the asthma is established, cycles of acute and chronic inflammation triggered by allergens, viruses, pollutants, diet and stress are responsible for exacerbations.

Recent studies indicate that the rise in childhood obesity may also be linked with the rise in childhood asthma. Children with high body mass indices were more likely to have symptoms of asthma, suggesting that increased weight might lead to a risk of inflammation in the respiratory tract or might hinder respiratory flow (Figure 11.7).

Primary preventative measures to reduce risk might therefore include allergen avoidance, cessation of smoking and attenuation of a Th2 response by vaccination. Once asthma is established, however, T cells and eosinophil responses may have enhanced capacity to generate the leukotrienes IL-3, IL-4 and IL-5 and it may be more difficult to reverse an established Th2 response. In this situation, secondary prevention measures to reduce exposure to trigger factors are appropriate.

Trigger factors in asthma

During the preschool years viral infections, exercise, and emotional upset are common triggers of asthma. Young children contract six

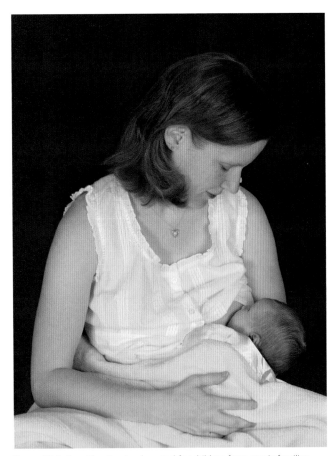

Figure 11.6 Breastfeeding is advocated for children from atopic families.

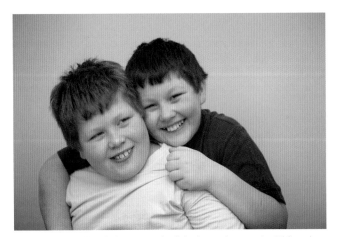

Figure 11.7 Childhood obesity may be linked to an increase in childhood asthma.

to eight viral upper respiratory tract infections each year; so it is not surprising that these infections are more common precipitants of asthma in children than in adults. Asthmatic children tend to have more symptoms during the winter than the summer, probably because viral respiratory infections are more common in winter and because exercise-induced asthma is more likely to develop outdoors in cold weather (Box 11.2).

Box 11.2 **Trigger factors in asthma**
- Viral infections
- Dusts and pollutants including cigarette smoke and diesel particulates
- Allergens – house dust mite, pollens, moulds, spores, animal dander and feathers, certain foods and *Alternaria* in dry arid conditions
- Exercise
- Changes in weather patterns and cold air
- Psychological factors such as stress and emotion

The domestic environment

If asthmatic children are sensitised to house dust mite, parents can reduce exposure by removing carpets or vacuum cleaning regularly and dusting surfaces with damp cloths, as well as encasing mattresses and pillows in plastic sheets, washing covers, blankets, duvets, and furry toys regularly, and applying acaricides to soft furnishings (Figure 11.8).

A recent Cochrane review (issue 4 2004), however, suggests that chemical and physical measures to reduce house dust mite cannot be recommended on the basis of present evidence.

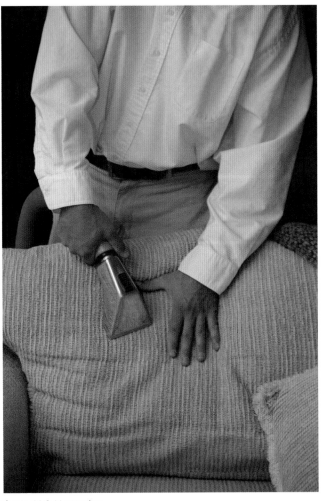

Figure 11.8 Vacuuming.

It must be borne in mind that intensive cleaning measures may also reduce the child's exposure to endotoxin and other bacterial components. Some studies indicate that early life exposure to cats and dogs may reduce the subsequent prevalence of asthma and allergy, giving further credence to the 'hygiene hypothesis.'

Smoking

Tobacco smoke has consistently been found to trigger exacerbation of asthma in children, and families should be encouraged to stop smoking or smoke in areas away from children outside the house. In addition, in families with a strong family history of asthma, and in children exposed to maternal smoking during pregnancy, there is a fourfold risk of developing wheezing illnesses in young children.

Studies have also demonstrated a decrease in asthma severity in children whose parents have ceased smoking (Figures 11.9–11.11).

Air pollution

Epidemiological studies have suggested that certain types of outdoor air pollution (sulphur dioxide and high diesel particulate

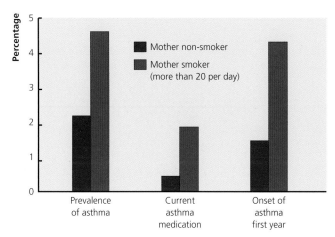

Figure 11.9 Maternal smoking and asthma in 4331 children aged 0–5, based on National Health Service (NHS) interview survey.

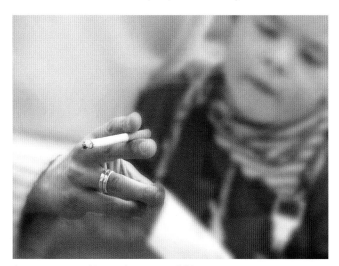

Figure 11.10 Smoking mother next to child.

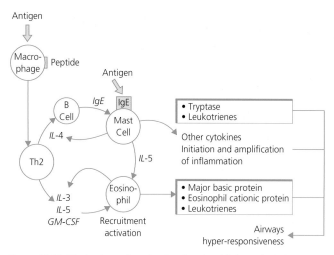

Figure 11.11 Mechanisms of mast cell and eosinophil-dependent airway hyper-responsiveness. Adapted from Drazen JM *et al. Journal of Expiratory Medicine* 1996; 183: 1–5.

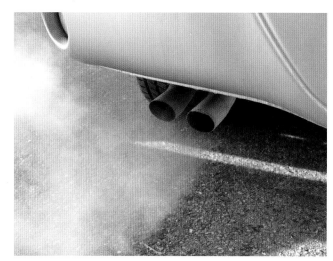

Figure 11.12 Diesel particles.

environment) may provoke emergency admissions for asthma or aggravate existing chronic asthma (Figure 11.12).

Indoor air pollution from gas stoves, for example, may prove to be a bigger culprit, and further research is required in this area.

Intervention

Tertiary prevention includes the provision of up to date guidelines to improve bronchodilation, reduce inflammation and improve quality of life. In addition, airway remodelling may occur early in the course of disease and may then lead to irreversible loss of pulmonary function. The early administration of topical steroids may modify this development, particularly in those with an allergic phenotype.

Airway inflammation and hyper-responsiveness

Airway hyper-responsiveness in young children can be assessed by a methacholine challenge test and a good clinical history and examination is probably a better diagnostic tool. However, a negative methacholine test in children has a high negative predictive value, that is, children are unlikely to have asthma with a negative challenge.

Indirect evidence of an inflammatory process in the airways of young children has come from measurement of markers of inflammation (e.g. eosinophils) in the blood and bronchoalveolar lavage, and measurement of exhaled nitric oxide concentrations (FE_{NO}). Higher sputum eosinophil counts are associated with atopy, airways obstruction and reversibility and a greater asthma severity. A higher FE_{NO} is more indicative of an atopic child with other atopic disorders (allergic rhinitis and eczema) than with asthma.

No component of the inflammatory process can be used as a diagnostic test for childhood asthma or as a reliable way to assess response to treatment. Diagnosis and the choice of treatment still depend on clinical judgement based on the nature, frequency and severity of symptoms combined with physiological assessment of airway function.

Further reading

Alm B, Aberg N, Erdes L *et al.* Early introduction of fish decreases the risk of eczema in infants. *Archives of Disease in Childhood* 2009; 94: 11–15.

Asher IM, Montefort S, Bjorksten B *et al.* Worldwide time trends in the prevalence of symptoms of asthma, allergic rhinoconjunctivitis, and eczema in childhood: ISAAC phases one and three repeat multicountry cross-sectional surveys. *Lancet* 2006; 368: 733–743.

Illi S, von Mutius E, Lau S *et al.* For the Multicentre Allergy Study (MAS) Group. Perennial allergen sensitisation early in life and chronic asthma in children: A birth cohort study. *Lancet* 2006; 368: 763–770 (with correction on page 1154).

Malmberg LP, Pelkonen AS, Haahtela T, Turpeinen M. Exhaled nitric oxide rather than lung function distinguishes preschool children with probable asthma. *Thorax* 2003; 58: 494–499.

Prasad A, Langford B, Stradling JR, Ho LP. Exhaled nitric oxide as a screening tool for asthma in school children. *Respiratory Medicine* 2006; 100 (10): 67–73.

Priftanji A, Strachan D, Burr M *et al.* Asthma and allergy in Albania and the UK. *Lancet* 2001; 358: 1426–1427.

Woodcock A, Lowe LA, Murray CS *et al.* Early life environmental control effect on symptoms, sensitization and lung function at age 3 years. *American Journal of Respiratory and Critical Care Medicine* 2004; 170 (4): 433–439.

CHAPTER 12

Patterns of Illness and Diagnosis

Dipak Kanabar

Evelina Children's Hospital, Guy's and St Thomas' Hospitals, London, UK

OVERVIEW

- It is important to distinguish between wheeze and upper airway noises
- The spectrum of childhood asthma distinguishes between transient wheezers, persistent wheezers and methacholine-responsive wheezers
- The goals of treatment for teenagers with asthma are psychological well-being, full physical activity and minimal effects on the underlying developmental progression from childhood to adulthood
- With appropriate explanation and reassurance about the condition, parental anxiety is more likely to be reduced and compliance with therapy increased

Wheezing in infancy

Wheezing is a high-pitched musical sound arising from the lower airways of the lung. It is important to distinguish this respiratory noise from stridor and stertor, which are upper airways noises.

As discussed earlier, young children up to the age of 5 are particularly prone to wheezing illnesses caused by rhinoviruses and respiratory syncytial virus. Researchers have differentiated early transient wheezers from persistent wheezers by analysis of risk factors and lung function tests. Transient wheezers had smaller airways and their mothers smoked, whereas the persistent wheezers had a more classical atopic history with a positive family history of maternal asthma, raised serum immunoglobulin E (IgE) levels and positive results to skin prick tests. A third group of children with transient symptoms which can sometimes persist into school age fall into the category of non-atopic wheezers. This latter group also show bronchial hyper-reactivity to methacholine (Figure 12.1) (Box 12.1).

Box 12.1 **Results of a prospective study by Martinez** *et al.* **(1995)**

A prospective study by Martinez and his colleagues in 1995 looked at over 1200 children born in Tucson, Arizona. By the age of 6,

---

826 children (51%) had never wheezed. Three patterns were identified in the others: 20% of children who had wheezed early on with respiratory tract infections had no wheezing by the age of 6 (early transient group), 15% had no wheezing at the age of 3 but had wheezing at the age of 6 (late onset group) and 14% had wheezing before the age of 3 and at the age of 6 (persistent wheezers).

Respiratory tract infections

Many young children have repeated episodes of wheezing associated with viral respiratory tract infections, and in particular, those who are suffering from or have had RSV bronchiolitis. These infections cause obstruction of the airways with desquamated airway epithelial cells, polymorphonuclear cells and lymphocytes. Recurrent cough and wheezing commonly follow, but in most cases stop before school age.

The mechanism by which this happens is still not fully understood, but genetic constitution and environmental influences in early life may predispose to wheeze by causing changes in airway calibre or lung function. For example, wheezy lower respiratory illnesses are more common among boys, among infants of parents who smoke and among babies born prematurely who have needed prolonged positive-pressure ventilation. Thus, pre-existing factors other than asthma that cause narrowing of the airways account for more than half of the wheezing developed by infants.

About 40% of babies with atopic eczema also develop recurrent wheezing and there is a strong association between a family history

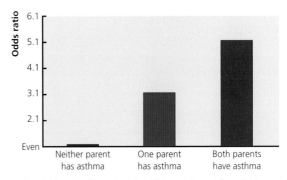

Figure 12.1 Odds ratios for asthma in children (adapted from Weitzman M *et al.*, *Pediatrics* 1990; 85: 505–511).

ABC of Asthma, 6th edition. By J. Rees, D. Kanabar and S. Pattani.
Published 2010 by Blackwell Publishing.

of atopic disease and wheezing in early childhood. According to Martinez's data, 14% of children had persistent wheezing from infancy to the age of 6 years (persistent wheezers), and this group also had the highest proportion of viral respiratory disease in the first year of life, suggesting that some viral infections may facilitate the development of asthma, whereas others (as discussed in Chapter 11) may help to modify the immune response in such a way as to protect against asthma.

Progression of asthma from childhood to adolescence

The outcome of early onset wheeze is still controversial. Children seen in referral centres have poorer outcomes than those followed up in longitudinal studies of general populations, probably because those with more severe asthma are referred to hospital.

Predictability

The data from Martinez and colleagues would suggest that early onset asthma is associated with poor outcome in terms of lung function and persistent bronchial hyper-responsiveness. Another study in infants aged 1 month showed that those who were more responsive to histamine challenge were more likely to have asthma diagnosed at the age of 6, and other studies have shown a clear relationship between degree of airway hyper-responsiveness to histamine challenge and persistence of asthma.

In a review of patients aged 29–32 who had previously been studied at the age of 7 by questionnaire and spirometry, however, Jenkins and colleagues found that of those who had reported asthma at age 7, only 26% had symptoms as adults. Other childhood risk factors which predict asthma in adult life include later onset of disease (aged over 2), female sex, a family history of asthma and more severe asthma at a young age.

A population study in New Zealand reported that as children grow older bronchial hyper-reactivity decreases. Judged by the response to inhaled histamine, the number of children with hyper-responsive airways halved between the ages of 6 and 12. In contrast, the total number of children with atopy doubled. Of those between the ages of 5 and 7 who had evidence of bronchial reactivity, about 50% were atopic; of the children aged 13 with bronchial hyper-responsiveness over 90% were atopic.

Results of studies

These results support the clinical observations that non-specific factors – notably viral infections and exercise – are important triggers of asthma during pre-school years and allergic triggers assume greater importance as children grow older. Other similar longitudinal studies suggest that children with mild disease usually outgrow their asthma as a result of the increase in airway size with growth and the apparent spontaneous decline in airway responsiveness with age. However, females and those with more severe disease, greater airway hyper-responsiveness and an atopic history have persistent disease.

Teenagers with asthma

Asthmatic teenagers are coping with a period of intense emotional and psychological change, and this can have a considerable impact on quality of life. They also have concerns about body image, peer acceptance, physical capabilities in terms of exercise and activity and physiological delay of puberty caused by their asthma, all of which can complicate their asthma treatment goals.

In addition, because of a need to emphasise their own identity, they may become isolated and may experience anxiety and depression, especially if they are excluded from participation in the decision-making process regarding their condition. They may also participate in risky behaviour such as cigarette smoking and non-compliance with treatment, which may account for their increased morbidity and mortality (Figure 12.2) (Box 12.2).

> Box 12.2 **The Goals of treatment for teenagers with asthma**
>
> The goals of treatment for teenagers with asthma are psychological well-being, full physical activity and minimal effects of the underlying developmental progression from childhood to adulthood.

The weekly incidence of acute asthma attacks diagnosed by a general practitioner increased markedly during the 1970s and 1980s, peaked in the early 1990s, and by 2000 declined quite substantially for the age groups of <5 and 5–14. Between 1990 and 2000, hospital admission rates had decreased by 52% among children under 5 years and by 45% among children aged 5 to 14 years.

These are all very encouraging statistics and suggest that perhaps greater awareness of the problem and better management guidelines have helped reduce the burden of disease for the population of UK teenagers and reduce the need for urgent consultation in general practice or admission to hospital.

Sympathetic consultation

Paediatricians need to recognise the needs of these vulnerable teenagers by spending more time listening to their needs, helping them make choices of treatment and negotiating a plan of action

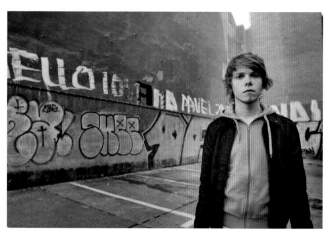

Figure 12.2 Asthma is often diagnosed in teenagers.

that allows for compromise on both sides. Holding separate clinics for young people and being prepared to discuss wider issues other than asthma may go some way to improve understanding and compliance.

Diagnosis of asthma

The diagnosis of asthma is made after an appropriate clinical history and examination, testing for reversibility of bronchoconstriction and assessing a response to therapy. Demonstrating airway reversibility or a short-term trial with anti-asthma therapy may be useful diagnostic markers, especially in those children with episodic symptoms (*see Chapter 3, p. 11*).

Presentation

In school-age children, there is little difficulty in recognising asthma, especially when one asks specifically about cough, wheeze, shortness of breath and exercise-induced symptoms. Pre-school children sometimes present with cough alone. The other characteristics that suggest asthma are episodic cough or wheeze, and symptoms worse at night, after exercise or exposure to allergens and with viral respiratory tract infections. Asthmatic babies sometimes have attacks of breathlessness without obvious wheezing.

Hypersecretory asthma

Some asthmatic children produce large amounts of bronchial secretions. This is called *hypersecretory asthma*. Increased production of mucus is associated with a productive cough, airway plugging and areas of collapse on the chest radiograph. These children may be misdiagnosed as having recurrent lower respiratory tract infection.

Most wheezing in infancy is due to accumulation of secretions in the airway in response to bronchial inflammation. However, certain features suggest that the cough or wheezing may be caused by conditions other than asthma. These factors include onset after birth, chronic diarrhoea or failure to thrive, recurrent infections, a persistent wet cough, stridor, choking or difficulty with swallowing, mediastinal or focal abnormalities on the chest radiograph and the presence of cardiovascular abnormalities (see Table 12.1).

Lung function and other tests

When possible, the diagnosis should be confirmed by lung function testing. This can be done at any age, but in infants and very young children the facilities are available only in specialised centres. From

Table 12.1 Other causes of noisy breathing in children.

• Bronchiolitis	• Laryngeal problem
• Inhalation – such as foreign body, milk	• Tuberculosis
	• Bronchomalacia
• Gastro-oesophageal reflux	• Tracheal/bronchial stenosis
• Cystic fibrosis	• Vascular rings
• Ciliary dyskinesia	• Mediastinal masses

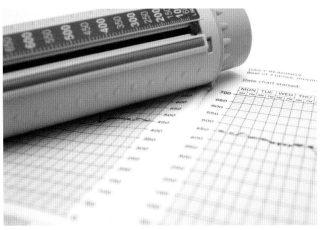

Figure 12.3 A peak flow metre can be used by some children (over 4 years) to test lung function.

the age of 4 years some children can use a peak flow meter, and the peak flow reading can be compared with a range of values related to the child's height. A normal peak flow reading at one examination does not exclude asthma, and several recordings made at home may be more valuable. If the result of spirometry is normal, then reversibility testing is of little use. Occasionally, an exercise test or therapeutic trial is necessary to confirm the diagnosis. Measurement of total IgE concentration will ascertain only whether the child is atopic. A chest radiograph is more useful to look for other causes of wheezing than to diagnose asthma (Figure 12.3).

Labelling

Making a diagnosis of asthma carries with it a certain stigma, for no parent likes to be told that their child may have a chronic illness with the possibility of recurrent exacerbations. However, with appropriate explanation and reassurance, parental anxiety is more likely to be reduced and compliance with therapy increased.

Assessment of severity

Ideally, the management of asthma should include serial measurement of markers of disease activity, but as yet, there are none which can be applied to the clinical care of asthmatic children. Evaluation of severity and response to treatment, therefore, has to be made by clinical assessment, complemented when possible by measurements of peak flow and lung function. A sound approach is to classify the asthma as mild, moderate or severe; to base the initial treatment regimen on this assessment; and then decide at regular reviews whether there is scope to modify medication.

Mild asthma

For asthma to be categorised as mild, symptomatic episodes should occur less frequently than once a month. Symptoms do not interfere with day-time activity or sleep. There is a good response to bronchodilator treatment, and lung function returns to normal between attacks.

Moderate asthma

Children with moderate asthma have some symptoms several days a week and have attacks of asthma more than once a month but less than once a week. There is no chest deformity and growth is unaffected. Attacks may be triggered by viral infection, allergens, exercise, cigarette smoke, climatic changes and emotional upset.

Severe asthma

The third category, severe asthma, is the least common. Children have troublesome symptoms on most days, wake frequently with asthma at night, miss school and are unable to participate fully in school or outdoor activities. They may be growth retarded and have chest deformities.

Some children do not fit into any of these categories. Seasonal asthma caused by allergy to grass pollen generally affects older children. A few children have sudden very severe attacks of asthma, which result in admission to hospital and may be life threatening, separated by long periods without symptoms during which their lung function returns to normal. This latter group are very difficult to treat.

Reference

Martinez FD, Wright AL, Taussig LM, Holberg CJ, Halonen M, Margan WJ. Asthma and wheezing in the first six years of life. The Group Health Medical Associates. *The New England Journal of Medicine* 1995; 332: 133–138.

Further reading

Asher IM, Montefort S, Bjorksten B *et al.* Worldwide time trends in the prevalence of symptoms of asthma, allergic rhinoconjunctivitis, and eczema in childhood: ISAAC phases one and three repeat multicountry cross-sectional surveys. *Lancet* 2006; 368: 733–743.

Custovic A, Simpson BM, Simpson A *et al.* Effect of environmental manipulation in pregnancy and early life on respiratory symptoms and atopy during the first year of life: a randomised trial. *Lancet* 2001; 358 (9277): 188–193.

Liu AH. Endotoxin exposure in allergy and asthma; reconciling a paradox. *Journal of Allergy and Clinical Immunology* 2002; 109: 379–392.

Sears MR, Green JM, Willan AR *et al.* Long term relation between breastfeeding and development of atopy and asthma in children and young adults. A longitudinal study. *Lancet* 2002; 360 (9337); 901–907.

CHAPTER 13

Treatment

Dipak Kanabar

Evelina Children's Hospital, Guy's and St Thomas' Hospitals, London, UK

OVERVIEW

- Asthma treatment should have clearly defined goals of therapy
- A stepwise approach to treatment is best for the patient
- A partnership arrangement should be encouraged
- Non-pharmacological therapies may have some benefit

There are several non-pharmacological therapies for the management of paediatric asthma, some of which have been discussed in earlier chapters. These include allergen avoidance measures and reduction of cigarette smoke exposure. Cochrane reviews (*The Cochrane library*) of other therapies, including complementary therapies, have shown some beneficial effect in the general well-being of the patient but no direct benefit in terms of asthma symptoms.

Pharmacological management

The aims of treatment are shown in Box 13.1.

Box 13.1 **Aims of treatment**

1. To control symptoms and allow children to lead a full and active life at home and at school
2. To restore normal lung function and reduce variations in peak flow
3. To minimise the requirement for bronchodilator therapy and prevent exacerbations
4. To enable normal growth and development and avoid adverse effects of medication

They can be achieved by prompt diagnosis, identification of trigger factors, evaluation of severity, establishment of a partnership of management with the asthmatic child and the family and regular review Box 13.2.

ABC of Asthma, 6th edition. By J. Rees, D. Kanabar and S. Pattani.
Published 2010 by Blackwell Publishing.

Box 13.2 **Outcomes of successful self-management**

1. Absence of or minimal cough, shortness of breath and wheeze, including nocturnal symptoms
2. Minimal or infrequent exacerbations
3. Minimal need for bronchodilator therapy
4. No limitation of activity, especially exercise and games
5. Restoration of normal lung function and reduction of variations in peak flow
6. Minimal or no adverse effects of the medications

Partnership in management

Self-management plans allow a partnership to be established between the doctor, the child and his or her family. The aim of the plan is to allow families to become more confident about the day-to-day management of asthma, to cope with exacerbations and to prevent hospital admission with early intervention and thereby ultimately reduce health costs. The goals of the partnership are listed in Box 13.3.

Box 13.3 **Goals of partnership**

1. An understanding of asthma and goals of treatment
2. Monitoring of symptoms
3. Use of a peak flow meter when appropriate
4. An agreed plan of action of what to do when the child's asthma improves, gets worse or there is an acute attack
5. Clear written instructions

In young children, plans are based on the child's symptoms and less so on objective assessments such as peak flow measurements. In older children, peak flow assessments are useful, especially for those who are poor perceivers of symptoms.

Respiratory nurses working in asthma clinics, schools and general practice play a pivotal role in establishing this partnership. They also keep regular personal contact and reassure and encourage children and their families. In addition, there is a wealth of information available from organisations such as Asthma UK.

Changing the environment

As mentioned earlier, the avoidance of cigarette smoking is important, especially during pregnancy. Families with asthmatic children should be discouraged from acquiring pets. With a pet already present, pet allergy has to be established with a good history of exacerbation following contact, as well as skin prick tests or specific immunoglobulin E (IgE) levels, before removal is advised. It may take several months before the animal dander completely disappears, and factors such as the emotional well-being of the child also have to be considered. There is some evidence, however, that maintaining a high cat-allergen exposure in the domestic environment might induce tolerance of the immune system.

House dust mite

House dust mite sensitivity is the most common allergy in asthmatic children. At high altitudes where concentrations of house dust mite and other inhaled antigens are low, symptoms, bronchial reactivity and the need for medication are considerably reduced.

However, only considerable environmental changes to reduce house dust mite have been shown to be effective in improving asthma Box 13.4.

Box 13.4 **Who are Asthma UK?**

Asthma UK is a charity dedicated to improving the health and well-being of people in the United Kingdom whose lives are affected by asthma.

Asthma UK produce useful leaflets for parents of newly diagnosed children and those who are living with asthma (available from website).

Website: www.asthma.org.uk

Advice line: 08457 01 02 03

Further reading

Platts-Mills T, Vaughan J, Squillance S *et al.* Sensitisation, asthma, and a modified TH2 response in children exposed to cat allergen: a population based cross-sectional study. *Lancet* 2001; 357: 752–756.

CHAPTER 14

Pharmacological Therapies for Asthma

Dipak Kanabar

Evelina Children's Hospital, Guy's and St Thomas' Hospitals, London, UK

OVERVIEW

- Most clinicians follow the BTS guidelines on management of childhood asthma
- It is important to monitor lung function at regular intervals
- It is important to monitor a child's growth during treatment with long-term steroids
- Refer to a specialist when there is uncertainty about the diagnosis or poor symptom control despite adequate therapy

The British Guideline on the Management of Asthma (2008) proposes a stepwise and algorithmic approach to drug management in paediatric asthma (Box 14.1).

Box 14.1 **Important points to remember when following the guidelines**

- There is a stepwise approach to asthma management for children aged 5–12 and children aged <5 years.
- Children should start at the step most appropriate to the severity of presentation of asthma and then move up or down the steps until a minimal effective dose of inhaled steroid is achieved to control symptoms.
- Before stepping up at any stage of treatment, ensure that compliance is good, that trigger factors are eliminated, that an appropriate inhaler device is given and that technique is good. Exclude other possible diagnoses such as gastro-oesophageal reflux, bronchiolitis, foreign body inhalation and cystic fibrosis.
- A rescue course of prednisolone at any step of 1–2 mg/kg/day is allowed for acute exacerbations for 3–5 days without the requirement for dose tapering. A short-acting bronchodilator can also be used more frequently during and after such exacerbations.
- Children with chronic asthma should be reviewed every 3–6 months and if they are stable, advised to reduce the dose of inhaled steroid by 25–50% until a minimum effective dose is achieved.

Inhaled short-acting β_2-agonists (bronchodilators)

Children with mild episodic asthma need only intermittent treatment with short-acting bronchodilator drugs, which should be given whenever possible by inhalation (Step 1 of the guidelines). Those with more severe asthma who are taking a prophylactic agent should always have a short-acting bronchodilator readily available. The selective β_2-adrenergic agonists (e.g. salbutamol and terbutaline) are the best and safest bronchodilators. Asthma in childhood is often triggered by viral respiratory tract infections and exercise. It may be necessary to take a bronchodilator as required during and for a week or two after a cold. A single dose of an inhaled β_2-adrenergic bronchodilator taken 15–20 minutes before a games period at school can also help to prevent exercise-induced wheezing.

Children with high usage of bronchodilator therapy more than three times a week should be reviewed with a view to consideration of additional preventative (prophylactic) therapy.

Prophylactic agents

The choice of prophylactic therapy depends on several factors, including drug efficacy, safety profile, ease of use and adherence to therapy. Topically active inhaled corticosteroids are very effective controllers of chronic asthma symptoms. Non-steroidal prophylactic agents include long-acting β_2-agonists, leukotriene antagonists and theophyllines (Box 14.2).

Box 14.2 **When to consider regular prophylactic medication**

- Frequent symptoms and the need to take a short-acting bronchodilator several days a week
- Frequent nocturnal cough and wheezing even without troublesome asthma during the day
- At least one asthma attack a month
- Lung function fails to return to normal between attacks

Lung function between attacks can be assessed by spirometric measurements of forced expiratory volume in 1 second (FEV1) and forced vital capacity (FVC). More subtle abnormalities can be detected by FEV curves or by measurement of lung volumes in a respiratory function laboratory.

ABC of Asthma, 6th edition. By J. Rees, D. Kanabar and S. Pattani.
Published 2010 by Blackwell Publishing.

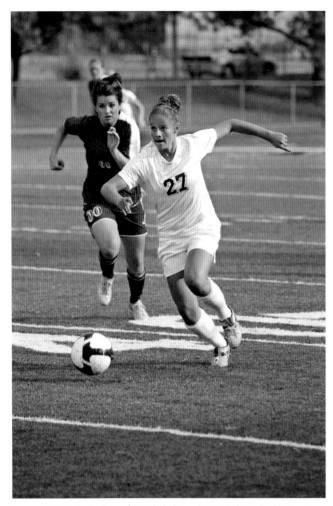

Figure 14.1 A single dose of an inhaled β₂-adrenergic bronchodilator can help to prevent exercise-induced wheezing.

A single measurement of peak expiratory flow rate (PEFR) may be misleading, but recordings made at home in the morning and afternoon or evening over a week or two may show variations that indicate airway instability and the need for prophylactic medication. Once started, regular treatment with a prophylactic agent is likely to be needed for years rather than months and should be withdrawn only when there has been little need for bronchodilator treatment for at least 3 months. Close supervision is necessary during withdrawal of a prophylactic drug (Figure 14.1).

Inhaled corticosteroids

Inhaled corticosteroids are an effective first-line prophylactic therapy for controlling asthma symptoms and improving quality of life (Step 2 of the guidelines), particularly in children aged over 5 years. In children aged less than 5, there may be a subgroup of children who are at high risk for asthma with an established history of recurrent wheezy episodes, a strong family history of asthma, allergy to an inhalant, atopic dermatitis and eosinophilia, who may also benefit from prophylactic steroid therapy.

It was believed that early introduction of inhaled corticosteroids may have prevented the progression of airways remodelling resulting from chronic inflammation; however, recent data suggests that inhaled corticosteroid therapy may after all not modify disease progression and prevent the development of episodic wheezing into persistent wheezing in children aged less than 5.

Dose

The starting dose depends on clinical assessment of severity, and in older children with frequent symptoms it may be appropriate to start with a moderate dose of inhaled corticosteroid, followed by reassessment of the patient to decide on add-on therapy. If control is successful with initial therapy, after a period of stability, steroid dose reduction to the minimum effective dose to prevent symptoms is recommended.

Current guidelines (2008) recommend a starting dose of 200–400 μg/day of beclomethasone diproprionate (BDP) or equivalent inhaled corticosteroid. The ceiling recommended dose is 800 μg/day, although higher doses can be used in some children to achieve early disease control.

Methods of delivery

When prescribed for the first time, children and their parents should receive adequate training in the use of the device and be able to demonstrate satisfactory technique. This ensures good drug delivery and reduces the likelihood of adverse effect.

Inhaled steroids given by pressurised aerosol (pressurised metered dose inhaler, (pMDI)), hydrofluoroalkane beclomethasone diproprionate (HFA-BDP) or by dry powder inhaler are effective in older children. The previous trend to use inhaled corticosteroids to treat asthma in children under 5 years, however, may be reducing as it is becoming increasingly recognised that many children with recurrent viral-induced wheeze do not go on to develop atopic asthma and probably would not benefit from long-term inhaled corticosteroid prophylaxis.

When it becomes necessary to prescribe an inhaled steroid to an under-5-year-old with frequent or severe asthma, pMDI and spacer with a one-way valve and a face mask is the best delivery system.

Adverse effects

There is a reluctance to give inhaled and oral steroids to young children because of a concern of possible side effects, and as a consequence long-term non-adherence to controller therapy is common in asthmatic children, with less than 50% of all prescribed doses taken.

Local side effects such as oral thrush and dysphonia are rare in children, probably because powder inhalers and spacer devices are used.

It is difficult to separate the adverse effects of asthma from the adverse effects of inhaled corticosteroids on children's growth. Likewise, if children whose asthma is well controlled on low-dose steroids are placed on high-dose steroids, growth may be stunted, whereas children with severe asthma may not experience any adverse effects but instead may enjoy a period of growth as a result of better control.

Evidence on the effects of inhaled corticosteroids on growth shows that both beclomethasone and budesonide at doses used at Step 3 or above of the British Thoracic Society (BTS) guidelines affect childhood growth as assessed by knemometry (leg length below the knee), and conventional stadiometry (Figure 14.2). Studies have not, however, shown any adverse effect on final height.

The exact mechanism of adverse of inhaled steroids on growth effect is unknown, but believed to be the result of decreased bone turnover, rather than that due to changes in growth hormone or IGF1 levels.

The effects of inhaled corticosteroids on bone mineral density are not proven. Long-term inhaled corticosteroids in boys may reduce bone mineral accretion in boys during puberty; however, it is the administration of multiple burst doses of oral steroids which has the greatest adverse effect on bone density.

A few children on high doses of inhaled corticosteroid have clinical adrenal insufficiency and present with hypoglycaemic episodes, coma or convulsions. Patients and parents have to be reminded of the dangers of stopping inhaled corticosteriods abruptly, and are advised to seek medical advice when such events occur.

Other studies suggest that the therapeutic gain at high doses of inhaled corticosteroids above 800 μg/day is likely to be small – the so-called ceiling effect, and therefore the clinician has to exclude other causes of treatment failure such as poor adherence to treatment and alternative diagnoses before using higher doses of inhaled corticosteroids as recommended at Step 4 of the guidelines (Figure 14.2).

Long-acting β_2-agonists

Long-acting β_2-agonists (LABA) are recommended as add-on therapy to inhaled steroids in adults and children aged >4 years at Step 3 of the BTS guidelines. In the United Kingdom, salmeterol is currently licensed for use in children from the age of 4 years, and formoterol in children over the age of 6 years. They increase airway calibre for at least 12 hours and prevent exercise-induced symptoms for up to 9 hours. The addition of LABA (salmeterol or formoterol) to the treatment of patients whose asthma is not well controlled on medium-dose inhaled corticosteroid improves lung function, decreases symptoms, reduces exacerbations and use of short-acting β_2-agonists.

Long-acting β_2-agonists are particularly useful for persistent nocturnal symptoms and troublesome exercise-induced symptoms. When control is not adequate at doses of inhaled steroid of 200 μg/day in children >5 years, add in a long-acting β_2-agonist first, together with the original dose of inhaled steroid. Thereafter if control remains poor, but there is benefit from addition of LABA, the dose of steroid can be increased up to 400 μg/day.

There has been a recent concern about the use of LABA, with report of an increased mortality in adult patients. Although there is no equivalent concern in paediatric practice, it is advisable to review patients regularly and monitor response to LABA add-on therapy. If patients report little or no benefit, then it is advisable to discontinue LABA use.

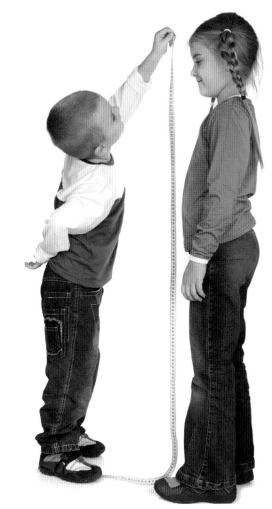

Figure 14.2 Stadiometry can be used to measure growth in children.

Leukotriene receptor antagonists

Leukotrienes released from mast cells and eosinophils mediate asthma by causing bronchoconstriction, mucous secretion and increased vascular permeability, promoting eosinophil migration into airways mucosa (Figure 14.3). Recent studies in children aged 6–17 have shown that children who have higher levels of allergic airways disease (with elevated levels of nitric oxide, raised immunoglobulin E (IgE) and eosinophil levels) are more likely to respond to inhaled corticosteroids than to leukotriene receptor antagonists (Box 14.3)

Box 14.3 When long-acting β_2-agonists are particularly useful

- When control is not adequate at doses of inhaled steroids >400 μg/day in children >5 years, add a long-acting β_2-agonist first, together with the original dose of inhaled steroid; the dose of steroid can then be increased up to 800 μg/day if control remains poor, in continuation with the long-acting β_2-adrenergic agonist.
- When children have persistent nocturnal symptoms and troublesome exercise-induced symptoms.

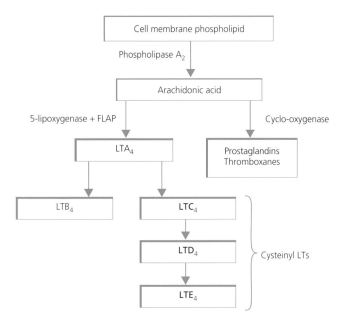

Figure 14.3 The leukotriene (LT) synthesis pathway. FLAP, 5-lipoxygenase activating protein.

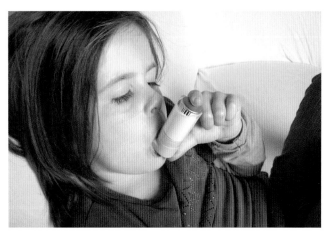

Figure 14.4 Child using a breath-actuated aerosol inhaler.

Leukotriene antagonists may be considered as an alternative to inhaled corticosteroids, where parents or their children are reluctant to take inhaled corticosteroids, or as adjunct therapy with inhaled corticiosteroids (Figure 14.4).

Currently in the United Kingdom, montelukast (available in granules or as a pink, chewable, cherry-flavoured tablet) is licensed for children over 2 years, and zafirlukast in those over 12 years of age.

Luekotrienes are currently used at Step 2 (children under 5 years) or Step 3 (children aged 5–12 years) in the management of paediatric asthma (Figures 14.5 and 14.6).

Omalizumab

Omalizumab is a monoclonal antibody that binds to the Fc portion of IgE antibodies preventing the binding of IgE to mast cells and basophils, leading to a reduction in the release of allergic mediators. It is licensed in children over 12 years with proven IgE-mediated sensitivity to aeroallergens (house dust mite, cockroach, cat or dog), whose severe persistent allergic asthma cannot be controlled adequately with high-dose inhaled steroids, oral steroids or a combination of inhaled corticosteroids and LABA. Its main disadvantages are that it has to be given by two weekly subcutaneous injection and there is a risk of anaphylaxis.

Several trials have shown clinical benefit with fewer exacerbations and a modest reduction in corticosteroid dose.

Magnesium

Low magnesium intakes have been associated with a higher prevalence of asthma, with increasing intake leading to reduced bronchial hyper-responsiveness and improved lung function. Its effect is likely to be mediated by bronchial smooth muscle relaxation.

Theophyllines

Theophylline can improve lung function and act as an effective bronchodilator with some anti-inflammatory action. Slow-release theophyllines in doses titrated to give blood concentrations of 10–20 mg/l will control asthma in children with frequent symptoms but they are relatively ineffective in preventing the wheezing which accompanies viral upper respiratory tract infections.

The variable clearance rate of theophylline means that it is difficult to predict the dose of the drug that will achieve therapeutic blood concentrations without causing toxicity. It is important to bear in mind that barbiturates, carbemazepine, phenytoin and rifampicin may reduce blood concentrations of thophylline and conversely cimetidine, erythromycin and ciprofloxacin may increase its concentration. Slow-release granule preparations may suit some children.

Side effects of theophyllines (notably gastrointestinal upsets and behaviour disturbances) are common, particularly in preschool children. Because of problems with giving the drug and its side effects, the use of theophyllines has been restricted to children whose asthma is uncontrolled despite treatment with inhaled steroids and where there has been no response to long-acting β_2-agonists and inhaled corticosteroid therapy.

Inhaler devices

Whenever possible asthma treatment should be given to children by inhalation, and the most common reasons for failure of inhaled treatment are inappropriate selection and incorrect use of the inhaler. Children become fully aware of their own breathing and recognise the difference between inspiration and expiration by about the age of 3; until then they need inhalation devices that require only tidal breathing. Inspiratory flow rates are slower and the airways narrower in children and both these factors influence the dose inhaled and the site of deposition of the drug. The choice of inhaler will depend on the child's age and preference for a particular device (Table 14.1).

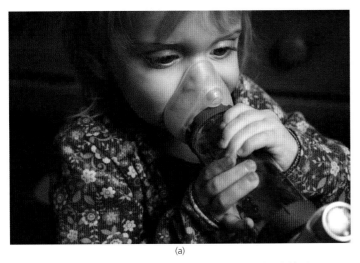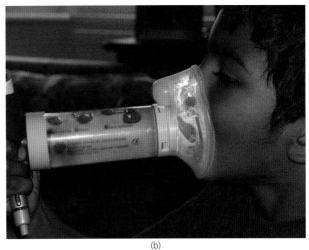

Figure 14.5 (a) Young child using an MDI and spacer. (b) Older child using an MDI and spacer.

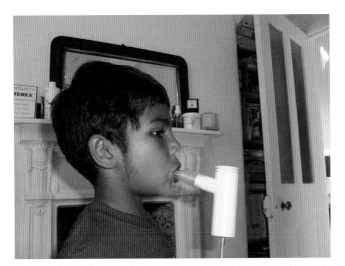

Figure 14.6 Nebulisers need to be used correctly in a domestic environment.

Table 14.1 Inhaler devices for children.

Age	1–2 years	3–5 years	>5 years
pMDI + spacer + mask	First choice	Second choice	–
pMDI + spacer	Second choice	First choice	Second choice
Breath-actuated MDI	Inappropriate	Useful	Equal first choice
Breath-actuated dry powder inhaler (DPI)	Inappropriate	Occasionally useful	Equal first choice

Aerosols and powders

Because of their detrimental effect on stratospheric ozone levels, chloroflurocarbon (CFC) propellants are being replaced by non-ozone depleting HFA propellants in pMDIs. Beclomethasone diproprionate with HFA pMDI has double lung delivery per dose actuation as beclamethsone diproprionate CFC pMDI and the dosages of HFA pMDI are correspondingly lower. Patients may also notice a slight taste difference when switched from CFC to HFA pMDI.

Most children under the age of 10 years are unable to achieve the coordination needed to use an unmodified pMDI. Less than half the children obtain benefit from these devices because of poor inhalation technique. Breath-actuated aerosol inhalers (Autohaler) are easier to use but children tend to close their glottis when the breath-actuated valve opens and fewer children under the age of 7 are able to use these inhalers.

The age at which breath-actuated dry powder inhalers such as the Accuhaler and Turbohaler can be used depends on the optimal inspiratory flow rate; for example, the Turbohaler needs an inspiration of about 30 l/min. The latter can therefore be used in children over the age of 4–5 years with proper training.

Spacers

A spacer device is an open tube placed at the mouthpiece of a pMDI to extend it away from the mouth of a patient. It works by reducing the velocity of the drug aerosol particles before they reach the mouth and allowing more of the propellant to evaporate so that the inhaled particles become smaller and penetrate further into the lungs. A parent actuates the pMDI device into the spacer, the child continues to breathe at tidal rate and thereby inhales the drug into the lungs.

A paediatric aerochamber, with a facemask in younger infants, is one of the most commonly used spacer devices. The spacer should be cleaned when it becomes cloudy and at least once a month. The spacer should be washed in soapy water and left to air dry. Where possible they should be replaced every 6–12 months.

Nebulisers

A Cochrane database systematic review updated in 2006 concluded that β_2-agonists pMDI therapy with a spacer is at least as good as a nebuliser at treating mild and moderate exacerbations of asthma. In wheezy infants short-acting β_2-adrenergic bronchodilators inhaled through a nebuliser may sometimes be associated with worsening of intrathoracic airway function: the poor response may be related to the small dose of drug reaching the airways or there may be a functional variability in response associated with polymorphisms of the β_2-receptor. In young children the anticholinergic agent ipratropium bromide may be beneficial, given either through a nebuliser or a spacer device with a facemask.

Nebulisers are expensive, time consuming and inconvenient. They are often used incorrectly at home. A compressor and jet nebuliser suitable for giving asthma medication should have a driving gas flow rate of 8–10 l/min and a volume fill of 4 ml. Despite these reservations, however, there is an important place for the judicious use of nebulisers in the treatment of young asthmatic children at home.

Choice of device

Patient preference is of major importance in the choice of device. Many children are unable to use pMDIs correctly and even with good technique, only 10–15% of the dose is delivered to the lungs.

Spacer devices will reduce coordination problems and improve lung deposition. Children on regular prophylactic inhaled steroids are advised to use a spacer at all times. Even when a spacer device is used, correct positioning of the device, inhalation of the drug within 10–20 seconds, single dose actuations, and regular rinse and drip drying of the spacer devices are important take home instructions.

Dry powder inhalers may also vary in their lung deposition, and up to 30% of a drug may reach the lungs with a good technique. The main determining factor for their use is variations in the inspiratory flow rate (Box 14.4).

Box 14.4 **When to refer to a specialist**

1. Uncertainty about the diagnosis
2. Poor symptom control despite adequate therapy within guidelines
3. Patient on high doses of inhaled steroid (above 800 μg/day)
4. Parental concern/request for a second opinion
5. Evidence of side effects

The future

Our understanding of the pathogenesis and classification of the subtypes of childhood asthma continues to improve. However, we still need to identify more precisely those factors that can prevent the onset of disease and modify disease progression. Genetic markers should enable us to identify those children at risk, as well as allow more specific pharmacological therapies in individual cases. Immunomodulation and modification of fetal and early life environmental factors are currently being evaluated, but in the meantime we need to improve both our and our patients' understanding of the disease, improve adherence to therapy and continue to follow guidelines of management in order to minimise the potential side effects of therapy.

Further reading

Allen DB, Bielory L, Derendorf H *et al*. Inhaled corticosteroids: past lessons and future issues. *Journal of Allergy and Clinical Immunology* 2003; 112: S1–S40.

Bisgaard H, Hermansen MN, Loland L *et al*. Intermittent inhaled corticosteroids in infants with episodic wheezing. *New England Journal of Medicine* 2006; 354: 1998–2005.

Guilbert TW, Morgan WJ, Zeiger RS *et al*. Long-term inhaled corticosteroids in preschool children at high risk for asthma. *New England Journal of Medicine* 2006; 354: 1985–1997.

Humbert M, Beasley R, Ayres J *et al*. Benefits of omalizumab as add-on therapy in patients with severe persistent asthma who are inadequately controlled despite best available therapy. *Allergy* 2005; 60 (3): 309–316.

Israel E, Chinchilli VM, Ford JG *et al*. Use of regularly scheduled albuterol treatment in asthma: genotype stratified randomised, placebo-controlled cross over trial. *Lancet* 2004; 364 (9444): 1505–1512.

Masoli M, Weatherall M, Holst S *et al*. Systematic review of the dose-response relation of inhaled fluticasone porprionate. *Archives of Disease in Childhood* 2004; 899: 902–907.

Medicines and Healthcare Products Regulatory Agency. Asthma: long-acting 2 agonists. Available at http://www.mhra.gov.uk/home/ . . . October 2009.

Nelson HS, Weiss ST, Bleecker ER *et al*. The Salmeterol Multicenter Asthma Research Trial: comparison of usual pharmacotherapy for asthma or usual pharmacotherapy plus salmeterol. *Chest* 2006; 129: 15–26.

Turner S, Thomas M, von Ziegenweidt J, Price D. Prescribing trends in asthma: a longitudinal observational study. *Archives of Disease in Childhood* 2009; 94: 16–22.

Walders N, Kopel SJ, Koinis-Mitchell D, McQuaid EL. Patterns of quick relief and long term controller medication use in paediatric asthma. *Journal of Paediatrics* 2005; 146: 177–182.

Zeiger RS, Szefler SJ, Phillips BR *et al*. Response profiles to fluticasone and montelukast in mild-to-moderate persistent childhood asthma. *Journal of Allergy and Clinical Immunology* 2006; 117 (1): 45–52.

CHAPTER 15

Acute Severe Asthma

Dipak Kanabar

Evelina Children's Hospital, Guy's and St Thomas' Hospitals, London, UK

OVERVIEW

- Keep a clear protocol at hospital or in your surgery of what steps to take in an emergency
- Decide early on whether the child warrants a hospital admission
- Ask parents/carers to keep an emergency card with a clear management plan

---

Parents and children need clear instructions about what to do when an acute asthma attack occurs and when to ask for medical help. Treatment should be initiated at home with a large dose of a β_2-agonist bronchodilator. Up to 10 puffs salbutamol or terbutaline by pressurised metered dose inhaler (pMDI) plus spacer with or without facemask with one puff given every 15–30 seconds or a nebulised bronchodilator therapy every 20–30 minutes is advised as a trial of therapy whilst the family seeks medical attention.

A child who responds well to a high dose of bronchodilator at home and who is not subsequently transferred to hospital will need to be reviewed a few hours later, and may require increased prophylactic treatment – either an increase in inhaled steroid therapy or a short course of oral prednisolone at 1–2 mg/kg/day.

If the child fails to respond or relapses despite the above management, oral prednisolone, regular β_2-agonist bronchodilator and oxygen should be given. Arrangements should also be made to transfer the child to hospital (Box 15.1 and Figure 15.1).

Box 15.1 **Indicators of acute severe asthma in children**

Child aged <5 years
- Child is too breathless to talk or feed.
- Child cannot complete sentences.
- Respiratory rate is >50 breaths per minute.
- Pulse rate is >140 beats per minute.
- The child uses accessory muscles.

Child aged ≥5 years
- Child is too breathless to talk or feed.
- Respiratory rate is >30 breaths per minute.
- Pulse rate is >120 beats per minute.
- The child uses accessory muscles.
- Peak flow is <50% best or predicted.

Oxygen and dehydration

Oxygen is important in treatment but sometimes difficult to give to toddlers. They become dehydrated because of poor fluid intake, sweating and, in the early stages, hyperventilation. This must be corrected, but there are potential risks of over-hydrating children with severe asthma. Production of antidiuretic hormone may be increased during the attack, and the considerable negative intrathoracic pressures generated by the respiratory efforts may predispose to pulmonary oedema. After correcting dehydration the wisest course is to give normal fluid requirements and measure the plasma and urine osmolality.

Steroids

Whilst a short course of oral prednisolone is widely used to treat preschool children with viral-associated wheeze, a recent randomised double-blind, placebo controlled study showed no benefit over placebo in mild to moderate cases.

Antibiotics

As most asthma attacks in childhood are triggered by viruses, and discoloured sputum is often due to inflammatory cells such as eosinophils and neutrophils, there is no role for antibiotics in the management of acute asthma.

Stabilisation

Children should not be discharged from hospital until they are taking the treatment that will be used at home and the peak flow rate is at least 75% of expected or best known.

A paediatric asthma nurse or a nurse experienced in this area should assess inhaler technique, give general advice and a written asthma action plan and arrange appropriate follow-up (Figure 15.2). This can improve the outcome and reduce the frequency of hospital readmission (Box 15.2).

ABC of Asthma, 6th edition. By J. Rees, D. Kanabar and S. Pattani. Published 2010 by Blackwell Publishing.

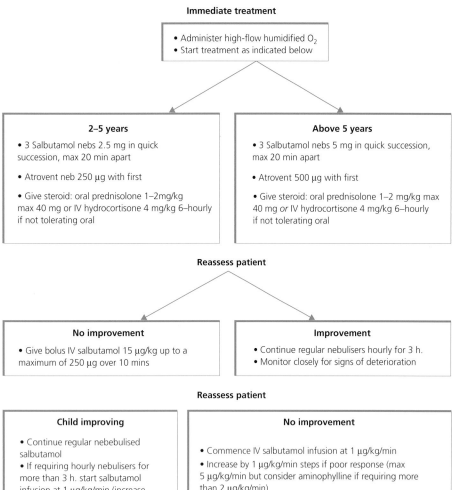

Figure 15.1 Management of acute severe asthma in children. CXR, chest X-ray; ECG, electrocardiogram.

Clinical signs to monitor severity and response to treatment

In young children it is often difficult to judge whether a particular treatment has had a beneficial effect, and clinical signs do not sometimes correlate with the severity of the attack.

Objective measurements and clear and accurate recording of clinical signs are therefore very important when evaluating treatment. The following clinical signs should be recorded on a regular basis – every 15 minutes until the patient is stable, then hourly.

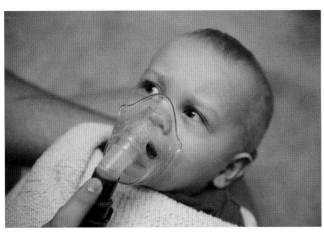

Figure 15.2 Nebulised therapy being given via mouthpiece during treatment for an acute episode of asthma.

1 Pulse rate: A tachycardia is usually seen in the acute phase of an asthmatic attack. Once the patient begins to respond to treatment, his or her heart rate reduces, but may increase again following β_2-agonist therapy. An increasing tachycardia generally indicates worsening asthma and a profound bradycardia may be a pre-terminal event.

2 Respiratory rate: Use of accessory muscles of respiration and subcostal recession are also useful markers of severity.

3 Degree of wheezing: Beware the silent chest! A child who does not wheeze with his or her acute asthma may have very limited airflow.

4 Glasgow Coma Score (modified paediatric).

Further reading

Panickar J, Lakhanpaul M, Lambert P *et al*. Oral prednisolone for preschool children with acute virus-induced wheezing *New England Journal of Medicine* 2009; 360 (4): 329–338.

CHAPTER 16

Clinical Aspects of Managing Asthma in Primary Care

Shriti Pattani

North West London Hospitals NHS Trust, and Hatch End Medical Centre, Harrow, Middlesex, UK

OVERVIEW

- Asthma produces significant morbidity and mortality with a prevalence of 5.4%
- An accurate diagnosis is the first step in reducing symptoms, functional limitations and impairment in quality of life
- The diagnosis is based on a good history and objective measures which demonstrate reversible airway obstruction using peak flow meter or spirometry
- Occupation is an important cause of asthma in the older patient. The type and nature of a patient's job is therefore an essential part of a complete history
- It is safe to continue with asthma medication during pregnancy and while breastfeeding
- The device chosen to deliver asthma medication must be matched to the patient's needs and abilities

Background

Asthma produces significant morbidity and mortality in the United Kingdom with a prevalence of 5.4% and 1200 deaths per year, some of which are preventable. Asthma costs the National Health Service (NHS) £1.0 billion per year (Asthma UK). General practitioners and practice nurses trained in asthma management are in a good position to monitor and educate patients regarding asthma control.

The natural history of asthma over time is either remission or increasing severity. The course of asthma usually varies between young children, older children, adolescents and adults. Young children can be particularly difficult to assess and treat.

Initial diagnosis

Making a diagnosis is the first step in reducing symptoms, functional limitations, impairment in quality of life and risk of adverse events that are associated with the disease. The diagnosis is based on a good history of variability in symptoms and peak flow/spirometry (Figures 16.1–16.3). Peak flow/spirometry is not routinely possible in children younger than 6 years so their clinical symptoms and signs must be carefully assessed.

ABC of Asthma, 6th edition. By J. Rees, D. Kanabar and S. Pattani.
Published 2010 by Blackwell Publishing.

History

Relevant points in the history are cough, particularly worse at night, recurrent wheeze, recurrent and episodic difficulty in breathing and chest tightness. The symptoms can occur at anytime but are generally worse at night. The symptoms often get worse with exercise. Ask about the pattern and severity of symptoms, as these tend to be highly variable and unpredictable.

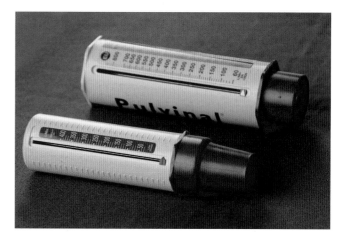

Figure 16.1 Adult and child peak flow meter.

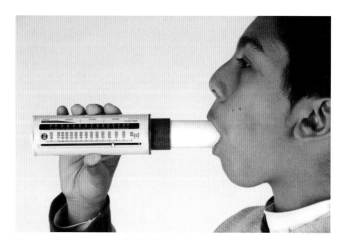

Figure 16.2 Important to check whether patient technique is optimal to produce an accurate reading (usually manageable in children aged 4 years and older).

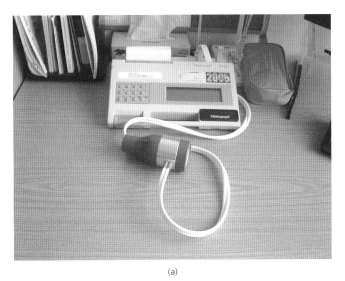

(a)

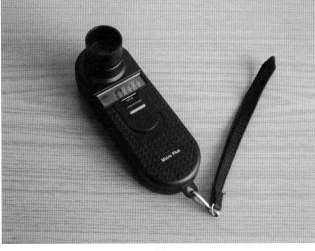

(b)

Figure 16.3 (a) Desk-top spirometer which is easy to use, store and transport and (b) portable hand-held spirometer which is easy to use in primary care.

Additional information which can be helpful include the following:

- Symptoms of blocked nose and sneezing; allergic rhinitis is very common among asthmatics.
- Ask about the relationship of symptoms to work, in particular whether they are better on days away from work.
- Ask about worsening of symptoms with the use of aspirin, nonsteroidal anti-inflammatory drugs (NSAIDs) and β-blockers.

Examination

Examination findings may be normal between exacerbations. In a patient who is short of breath the following should be checked:

- Patient's ease of communication, degree of shortness of breath, colour, chest movement and intercostal recession
- Respiratory rate, pulse rate, blood pressure, oxygen saturation (if pulse oximeter available), peak flow or spirometry
- Auscultation

Diagnosis

To confirm a diagnosis of asthma, objective measurements are used to demonstrate reversible airways obstruction. One of the following criteria needs to be fulfilled.

- More than 20% diurnal variation on at least 3 days a week for 2 weeks, as recorded in a peak flow diary (Figure 16.4)
- More than 20% improvement in peak expiratory flow rate (PEFR) or 15% and 200 ml improvement in forced expiratory volume in 1 second (FEV1) 10 minutes after inhalation of a short-acting β₂-agonist
- More than 20% deterioration after challenge with a trigger factor, for example, exercise

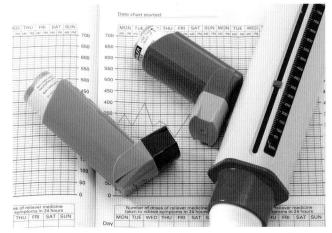

Figure 16.4 Peak flow diaries with accurate recording can assist in the diagnosis.

Diurnal variation (%) is calculated by

$$\frac{\text{Highest PEFR} - \text{Lowest PEFR}}{\text{Highest PEFR}} \times 100$$

Differential diagnosis

The following conditions can share similar symptoms to asthma in adults and therefore need to be considered in the list of differentials:

- Chronic obstructive pulmonary disease
- Laryngeal, tracheal and lung cancer
- Sarcoidosis
- Bronchiectasis
- Interstitial lung disease

Differentiation comes through a careful history and examination, spirometry to distinguish restrictive and obstructive problems, a chest x-ray or a chest clinic referral if the diagnosis is still in doubt.

Table 16.1 Step-up and step-down approach to manage pharmacological treatment.

	<5 years	5–12 years	12 years onwards
Device	pMDI* with a suitable spacer device with a face mask if required	pMDI* with a suitable spacer. If unable or unwilling use DPI or breath-actuated MDI	pMDI* with or without a spacer or DPI**
Step 1	Short-acting β₂- agonist	Short-acting β₂- agonist	Short-acting β₂-agonist
Step 2	Inhaled corticosteroids (ICS) if • having symptoms three times weekly or more; • awakening with symptoms one night weekly or more; • having an exacerbation in the last 2 yr; • using inhaled β₂- agonist three times weekly or more; • if ICS not tolerated or are contraindicated consider starting leukotriene receptor antagonist at this step (but only in children over 2 yr).		
Step 3	If symptoms persist despite regular ICS 2 years or under refer – Step 4 2–5 years – trial of leukotriene antagonist or refer Step 4	Consider starting long-acting β₂- agonist (LABA) if symptoms are still uncontrolled with ICS • If good response to LABA continue with current dose of corticosteroid • If good response but control still inadequate, continue LABA and ensure that inhaled corticosteroid dose is 400 μg in a child or 800 μ/d in an adult; if still inadequate move to Step 4 • If response to LABA is inadequate stop treatment and try an alternative leukotriene receptor antagonist or theophylline or go to Step 4	
Step 4	Refer to paediatrician	Consider increasing ICS up to 800 μg daily or Step 5	If control is still inadequate increase ICS to maximum dose (for beclomethasone – 2000 μg/d). If control remains, poor, consider adding leukotriene receptor antagonist or theophylline or oral modified-release β₂-agonist
Step 5		Refer to paediatrician	Refer to respiratory physician

*Pressurised metered dose inhaler.
**Dry powder inhaler.

Management

1 Use the step-up and step-down approach (Table 16.1) to manage pharmacological treatment using the most appropriate delivery system (Figures 16.5–16.9).

2 Explain the difference between reliever and preventer, discuss inhaler technique, trigger factors and self-management plan. Refer to nurse-led asthma clinic for a comprehensive follow-up and detailed self-management plan (see Chapter 17).

3 Provide lifestyle advice as appropriate such as weight reduction and support to stop smoking including the use of any local support networks that are available. Discuss vaccinations including those for influenza and pneumococcal disease.

4 Follow-up intervals can be yearly for a patient with well-controlled asthma although after initial diagnosis or following

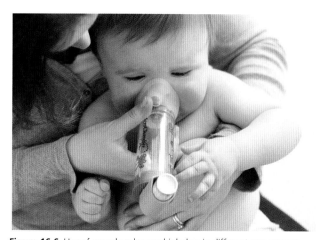

Figure 16.6 Use of aerochamber and inhalers in different age groups: childhood asthma. Mother helping her baby son to use an inhaler. The inhaler is attached to a spacer. The spacer acts as a reservoir, retaining the vapour from the inhaler and allowing the patient to inhale it at their chosen rate. RUTH JENKINSON/SCIENCE PHOTO LIBRARY.

an exacerbation more frequent review may be required. During the review assess asthma control including symptom control, medication review, lifestyle changes and self-management education.

Triggers

The following trigger factors need to be considered in the assessment:

- Respiratory infections
- Allergens, for example, house dust mites, pollen and furry animals
- Weather changes

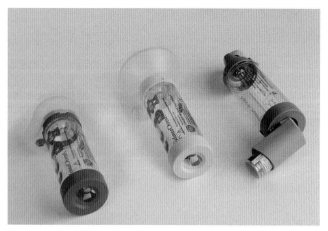

Figure 16.5 Aerochambers for infants and children with a mask and for the older child/adult.

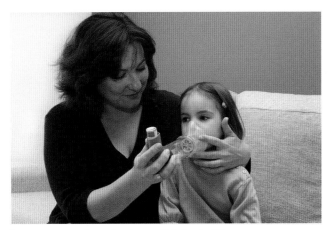

Figure 16.7 Use of aerochamber and inhalers in different age groups: aerochamber with a mask being used in a child with parental support.

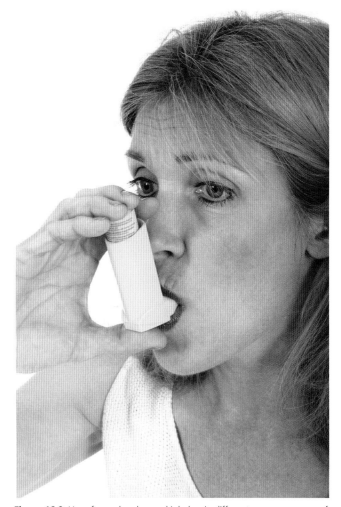

Figure 16.9 Use of aerochamber and inhalers in different age groups: use of an inhaler in an adult.

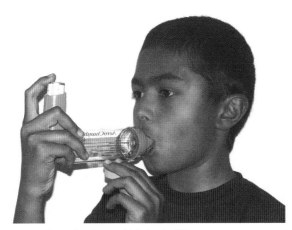

Figure 16.8 Use of aerochamber and inhalers in different age groups: use of an aerochamber without a mask in an older child.

- Exercise
- Emotional factors
- Gastro-oesophageal reflux disease
- Allergic rhinitis and sinusitis
- Drugs, for example, β-blockers and NSAIDs
- Occupational sensitisers, for example, isocyanates

Referral to secondary care

The following features warrant consideration of a referral to secondary care:

- The diagnosis is unclear
- Suspicion of occupational asthma
- Inadequate response to maximum guidelines treatment
- Non-resolving pneumonia
- Poor control of asthma symptoms despite optimal treatment

Occupational asthma

Nine to fifteen percent of asthma in older patients is related to occupation.

Take a history with particular reference to symptoms related to work, e.g. better on days away from work or on holidays. Occupations at high risk are those of paint sprayers, bakers, pastry makers and animal handlers.

Refer the individual to a respiratory specialist and in the meantime, ask them to keep a detailed peak flow diary, recording their peak flow ideally 2 hourly for 1 month, covering periods at and away from work. Advice and record forms are available on the website http://www.occupationalasthma.com.

Asthma, pregnancy and breastfeeding

There are no adverse maternal or fetal complications if asthma is well controlled during pregnancy. Uncontrolled asthma can cause complications such as hyperemesis, hypertension, pre-eclampsia, intrauterine growth retardation and neonatal hypoxia (Schatz *et al.*, 1995; Cydulka *et al.*, 1999). Primary care clinicians have an essential role in optimising asthma care and providing pre-pregnancy counselling for asthmatic patients including dangers of smoking and appropriate support to stop smoking.

It is safe for pregnant and breastfeeding females to continue their asthma medication (Figure 16.10). It is important that asthma

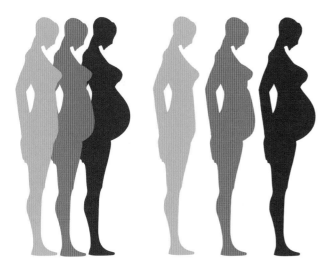

Figure 16.10 Optimising asthma control in pregnancy is essential to minimise complications. Asthma medication is considered safe in pregnancy.

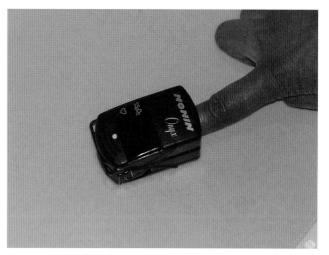

Figure 16.11 Use of a pulse oximeter is useful in the clinical assessment of patients with asthma in primary care; the device is easy to use and maintain.

treatment is optimal during pregnancy and preferably administered by inhalation to minimise exposure of the fetus. However, oral and intravenous (IV) theophyllines and oral steroids should be used as normal when indicated during pregnancy for severe asthma. Leukotriene receptor antagonists have not been shown to be safe during pregnancy. They should not be started during pregnancy but if already used and considered essential they should be continued. Provided the asthma is well controlled during pregnancy, there are no significant effects on pregnancy, labour or the fetus. Whilst breastfeeding, inhaled drugs, theophylline and prednisolone can be taken as normal.

Acute asthma

It is important to accurately assess the severity of symptoms, which will provide further information for a management plan. Symptoms will include cough, shortness of breath and chest tightness. Examination should include signs of exhaustion, cyanosis (bluish lips or extremities), respiratory rate, pulse, blood pressure, auscultation of the chest and peak flow recording if the patient is able to blow, using the best of three recordings to grade the severity of the attack on the basis of the best or predicted value. If a pulse oximeter is available measure the patient's oxygen saturation on room air (Figure 16.11).

Life threatening

Features of a life-threatening attack of asthma that can be recognised in general practice are as follows:

- Silent chest
- Cyanosis
- Confusion
- Exhausted slow respiration, bradycardia and hypotension
- PEFR <33% best or predicted

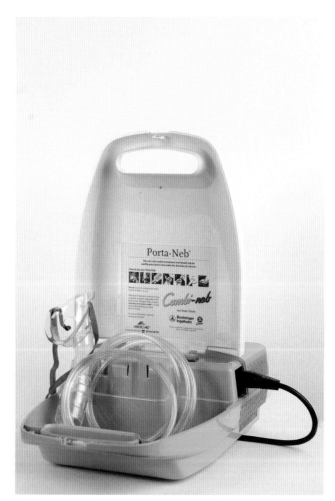

Figure 16.12 Nebulisers are easy to use, store and maintain in primary care.

Identification of any of the above features needs urgent management:

- Arrange immediate hospital admission.
- Give high-flow oxygen (40–60%) with a tight-fitting mask.

- Give an inhaled β_2-agonist via a nebuliser if available and ideally driven by oxygen.

If the patient is not responding, consider continuous nebulised β_2-agonist and the addition of nebulised ipratropium (Figures 16.12–16.13).

- If a nebuliser is not available use multiple doses of inhaled β_2-agonist via a spacer device.
- Oral steroid 40–50 mg or IV hydrocortisone.

Stay with the patient until the ambulance arrives.

Severe attack

Characteristic features of a severe attack are as follows:

Cannot complete sentences
Respiratory rate $\geq$25 breaths per minute
Pulse rate $\geq$110 beats per minute
PEFR 33–50% (best ever or predicted)
Oxygen saturation $\leq$93%

Moderate attack

Peak flow >50–75% of predicted or best
No features of acute severe asthma

Treatment of severe/moderate asthma

- High-flow oxygen if available
- Salbutamol or terbutaline via a large volume spacer (4–6 puffs, each inhaled separately; repeated every 10–20 minutes according to clinical response) or via nebuliser (although this is no more effective than an inhaler and spacer)
- Oral prednisolone 40–50 mg daily for at least 5 days
- Monitoring of response 15–30 minutes after nebulisation
  - If any signs of acute asthma persist or develop then arrange hospital admission.
  - If symptoms improve, respiration and pulse settle and peak flow is >50% of predicted or best peak flow, then step up usual treatment and continue prednisolone for at least 5 days.
  - The threshold for hospital admission should be lower if there has been a previous near-fatal attack or brittle asthma, pregnancy, presentation at night or in the afternoon, patient under 18 years, poor concordance or social circumstances.
- Treat any precipitating factors such as hayfever, bacterial infection and gastro-oesophageal reflux
- Follow-up
  - For severe asthmatics review within 24 hours.
  - For moderate asthmatics review within 48 hours.
  - In both cases it is important to review the cause of any exacerbation, the action followed and to ensure that patients understand an agreed asthma action plan.

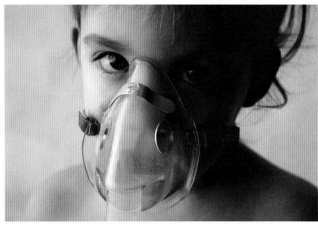

(a)

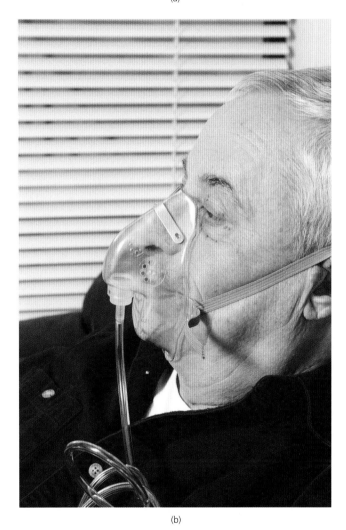

(b)

Figure 16.13 Nebuliser use in primary care can be useful for all age groups: (a) in children and (b) in adults.

References

Asthma UK. www.asthma.org.uk.

Cydulka RK, Emerman CL, Schreiber D, Molander KH, Woodruff PG, Carmargo CA Jr. Acute asthma among pregnant women presenting to the emergency department. *American Journal of Respiratory and Critical Care Medicine* 1999; 160 (3): 887–892.

Schatz M, Zeigler RS, Hoffman CP *et al*. Perinatal outcomes in the pregnancies of asthmatic women: a prospective controlled analysis. *American Journal of Respiratory and Critical Care Medicine* 1995; 151 (4): 1170–1174.

Further reading

British guideline on the management of asthma. http://www.brit-thoracic.org.uk/Portals/0/Clinical%20Information/Asthma/Guidelines/asthma_final2008.pdf *Thorax* 2008; 63 (Suppl IV).

CHAPTER 17

Organisation of Asthma Care in Primary Care

Shriti Pattani

West London Hospitals NHS Trust, and Hatch End Medical Centre, Harrow, Middlesex, UK

OVERVIEW

- Asthma care is greatly improved when delivered by doctors and nurses appropriately trained in asthma management
- The aim of asthma care is to achieve maximum control of the disease
- A structured planned approach with a written asthma plan achieves the best outcome for patients
- Organisation of asthma care requires an asthma register, practice protocol including process for diagnosis, treatment and referral criteria based on current guidelines agreed with the primary care team
- The Royal College of Physicians (RCP) three morbidity index questions can help to assess asthma control
- A personalised asthma plan can empower a patient to achieve very good asthma control on the lowest effective treatment with minimal side effects

The quality of asthma care given to patients in primary care is greatly improved when delivered by doctors and nurses who are trained in asthma management (Feder *et al.*, 1995; Clark *et al.*, 1998). The identified improvements relate to diagnosis, prescribing, monitoring and continuity of care based on current guideline levels. In 2001, the National Asthma Campaign identified that only one in four patients with a diagnosis of asthma had contact with a practice nurse and doctor.

Healthcare professionals often concentrate on end points such as lung function or the need to use reliever therapy as part of an assessment for degree of asthma control. However, patients' perception of good disease control is usually based on whether they are able to do the things they want to do. Current guidelines combine these two approaches, supporting the use of composite measures of asthma control.

The main factor in determining the outcome for patient care is being attended by clinicians appropriately trained in asthma management rather than whether a practice nurse or general practitioner conducts the review (Feder *et al.*, 1995; Dickinson *et al.*, 1997; Lindberg *et al.*, 1999). In the United Kingdom, it has been

shown that asthma-related morbidity improves significantly with a nurse-led asthma clinic leading to an improvement in patient's lifestyle (Charlton *et al.*, 1991).

The aim of asthma care

Patients' definition of good asthma control can be variable. Surveys have demonstrated that more than 66% of asthma patients who described their asthma as being 'under control' experienced symptoms at least two to three times a week (Haughney *et al.*, 2001). The goal in asthma care is to achieve maximum control of the disease (BTS/SIGN 2008). Control is defined as follows:

- No day-time symptoms
- No night-time awakening due to asthma
- No need for rescue medication
- No exacerbations
- No limitations on activity including exercise
- Normal lung function (in practical terms forced expiratory volume in 1 second FEV1 and/or peak expiratory flow PEF > 80% predicted or best) with minimal side effects.

Asthma clinics

A structured, planned approach to clinical review as opposed to opportunistic or unscheduled assessment achieves the maximum benefit, especially if it includes a discussion and the use of a written asthma plan (Figure 17.1). The benefits include a reported improvement in symptoms matched by objective measurements, reduced exacerbations, improvement in attendance at work and school and a reduction in days lost from normal activity (Feder *et al.*, 1995).

Some patients will not attend planned reviews and these individuals will clearly benefit from an opportunistic review. The content and discussion within the consultation determines the outcome of the assessment and is independent of whether the review was planned or opportunistic (BTS/SIGN, 2008). Therefore, it is important to have a structured approach with a standardised template for recording information which is used by all clinicians within the practice.

Telephone consultations to review asthma care may be as effective as face-to-face consultations (Pinnock *et al.*, 2003), particularly in

ABC of Asthma, 6th edition. By J. Rees, D. Kanabar and S. Pattani.
Published 2010 by Blackwell Publishing.

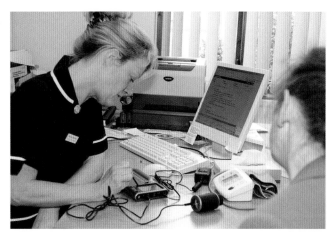

Figure 17.1 Healthcare professionals trained in asthma care can achieve better patient outcome. Lung function test. Nurse checking a patient's lung function test results. The patient has just breathed into a peak flow meter (spirometer) which measures the amount and speed of air that is exhaled. This is an important test for assessing conditions such as asthma, cystic fibrosis, and chronic obstructive airway diseases (COAD) such as bronchitis and emphysema. To view the patient blowing into the peak flow meter, see Fig. 17.2. LIFE IN VIEW/SCIENCE PHOTO LIBRARY.

those who are well controlled. It would be essential to undertake face-to-face review for those whose asthma control is poor or those who have inhaler-related problems.

Asthma register

The first important step in primary care is to have an established register of patients with asthma and an annual recall programme. In the United Kingdom, general practitioners are awarded points under the Quality and Outcomes Framework for aspects of asthma care. This forms part of their contract and translates into financial reward. Points are awarded for maintaining an asthma register, initial diagnosis based on set criteria and annual review. The register needs to be kept up to date and the practice protocol needs to define how this is going to be done.

Practice protocol

It is important that a clear protocol is available to clinical staff in the practice, which sets standards of care and allows auditing of the process. Ideally, the protocol needs to be jointly produced by a doctor with an interest in asthma and a nurse trained in asthma who will lead the clinics. The protocol needs to be based on current guidelines and agreed upon with the primary care team. The protocol needs to define processes for diagnosis, treatment plan and referral criteria either between doctor and nurse or to secondary care and review intervals. A review date for the protocol should also be set.

Initial assessment in asthma clinic

A structured approach focusing on subjective and objective measures of asthma control and expectation is important.

Subjective assessment

The three morbidity index questions recommended by the Royal College of Physicians to assess symptoms of asthma in the past week or month provides an appropriate assessment of control:

- 'Have you had your usual asthma symptoms during the day, such as cough, wheeze, chest tightness or breathlessness?'
- 'Have you had any difficulty sleeping because of your symptoms, including cough?'
- 'Has your asthma interfered with your usual activities (such as housework, job or school)?'

Other relevant information includes the following:

- Medical history
- Asthma history, both past and current
- Trigger factors
- Allergies
- Current asthma medication and any other medication, especially β-blockers, aspirin and nonsteroidal anti-inflammatory drugs (NSAIDs)
- Smoking history
- Occupational history.

Objective assessment

- Peak flow measurement, both predicted and best
- Spirometry (Figure 17.2a,b,c)
- Assessment of inhaler technique.

Other relevant measurements are as follows:

- Height
- Weight.

Personalised asthma plan

On the basis of discussion of the current situation and the understanding and expectations of the patient a personalised asthma plan should be produced. This should include the following:

- Nature of the disease
- Details of asthma drugs including names, doses, how to use and side effects; advice about when to take further action (for example, based on the pattern of their symptoms or peak flow measurements) (Figures 17.3 and 17.4)
- What to do if symptoms get worse
- When to return to usual doses
- When to seek urgent medical help.

The aim of treatment as supported by current guidelines is to maintain complete or very good asthma control on the lowest effective treatment with minimal or no side effects. A personalised plan will allow this stepping up and down according to symptoms and asthma history and also allow the patient to take charge of their symptoms. This may be supported by peak flow measurements.

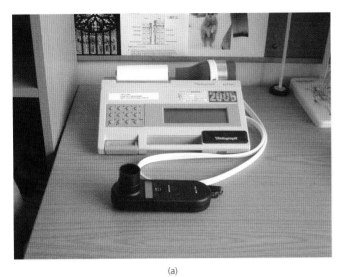

(a)

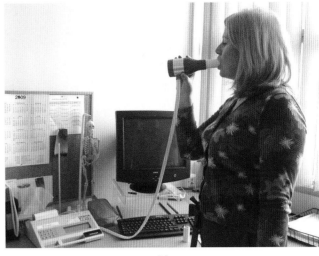

(b)

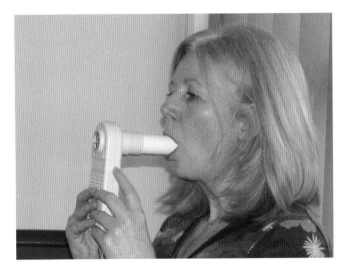

(c)

Figure 17.2 (a and b) Spirometer which produces a print out of the results. (c) Hand-held spirometer (no print out).

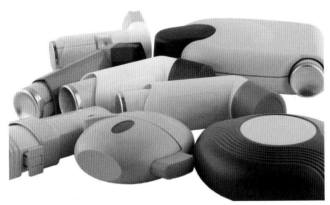

Figure 17.3 There is a variety of delivery systems. Choosing an inhaler which the patient can use with ease is essential in managing and controlling symptoms.

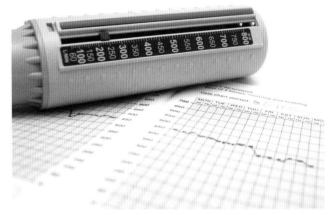

Figure 17.4 Peak flow measurements can empower patients in managing their treatment.

The personalised plan should also include an emergency management programme according to BTS/SIGN guidance, for example:

- If peak flow falls to XXX l/min (<50–75% of predicted), use a spacer to administer salbutamol or terbutaline (4–6 puffs each inhaled separately), repeat after 15–20 minutes and contact your doctor.
- If peak flow falls to XXX l/min (33–50% of predicted) and particularly if unable to talk in sentences, use a spacer as above and call for an ambulance.
- If peak flow drops below XXX l/min (33% of predicted), arrange immediate hospital admission; while waiting for an ambulance, use a volumatic as above.

Check the smoking status of the patient and advise on cessation if necessary. Recommend the influenza immunisation yearly and the pnuemoccocal vaccination. Organise a review appointment.

Review appointments

Generally patients with asthma need to be reviewed annually; however, the following category may benefit from more frequent reviews:

- Newly diagnosed
- Recently admitted to hospital or attended Accident and Emergency
- Recently treated with a course of oral steroids
- Frequent use of short-acting β_2-agonist (the equivalent of 1 or more prescriptions per month)
- Change in treatment.

The content of a review appointment should include the following:

- Symptom review based on the three RCP questions as outlined above
- Compliance with medication by direct questioning and prescription history
- Reviewing any concerns
- Reviewing medication
- Observing inhaler technique (Figure 17.5)
- Measuring peak flow (best of three)
- Checking smoking status and advise smokers on cessation
- Advising on annual influenza vaccination
- Ensuring that patient has a self-management plan and update as necessary
- Suggesting a suitable time interval for review.

Compliance

Obstacles to good symptom control include a failure to take medication, a poor understanding of asthma, why their treatment works, how to take their treatment, incorrect use of inhaler devices and anxieties about side effects and loss of effectiveness of regular treatment. Studies in Canada and Europe have revealed a lack of understanding of the role of corticosteroids and consequent under-use (Jones *et al.*, 2002).

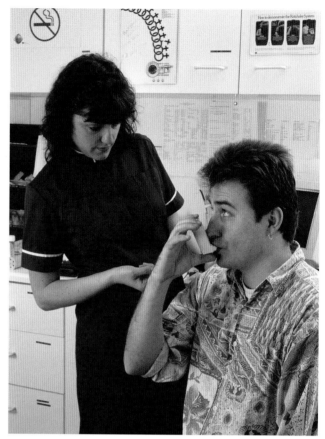

Figure 17.5 It is essential to check that the patient's inhaler technique is correct. Nurse instructing a young man (an asthma patient) in the use of a Becotide (R) inhaler. The Becotide inhaler contains the corticosteroid drug beclomethasone dipropionate. The action of corticosteroids in asthma is not fully understood, but it is believed they give relief by reducing inflammation in the bronchial mucous membrane, causing less oedema (fluid retention) and hypersecretion of mucous. Becotide aerosol inhalers deliver a dose of 50 or 100 micrograms (depending on type) per puff. A typical daily dosage using the lower strength inhaler would be 200 micrograms (4 puffs) twice daily. HATTIE YOUNG/SCIENCE PHOTO LIBRARY.

Compliance can be improved by good communication and involving patients in decision-making, which encourages them to take ownership of their self-management plans. Patients should be offered self-management education, which focuses on their individual needs reinforced by simple, verbal and written information.

The BTS/SIGN 2008 recommends the following to improve compliance:

- Ask open-ended questions like 'if we could make one thing better for your asthma what would it be?'
- Make it clear that you are listening and responding to the patients concerns and goals.
- Reinforce practical information and negotiate treatment plans with written instruction.
- Consider reminder strategies.
- Recall patients who miss appointments.

Auditing asthma clinic

The effectiveness of the clinic needs to be assessed in terms of both process and outcome. The aim of auditing is to demonstrate what works and identify areas of improvement. Examples of areas of suitable audit are as follows:

- Percentage of patients on the practice asthma register who are seen at least annually for a review
- Percentage of patients on the practice asthma register who have had their inhaler technique checked
- Percentage of patients on the practice asthma register who have a self-management plan
- Percentage of patients on the practice asthma register who are using regular treatment
- Number of patients requiring emergency visit or admission
- Number of clinicians who have taken part in suitable educational update within the last 2 years.

Criteria for referral to secondary care

The practice protocol needs to identify individuals who would be suited to refer to secondary care. As a guide, an adult whose occupation may be causing or contributing to their asthma, or those not responding to treatment despite being managed at step 4 of BTS/SIGN guidelines should be referred. Among children under 5 years referral is appropriate at an earlier stage (Step 3).

Training and support

Outcomes for patients are significantly improved if their asthma care is managed by clinicians trained in asthma management. The training methods identified as being successful include interactive education based on clinical guidelines and feedback from audit data on the clinical management of individual patients relative to current guidelines (Gibson and Wilson, 1996; Clar et al., 1998; Premarante et al., 1999). Therefore, time, money and appropriate training including mutual peer group support for doctors and nurses will need to be identified in primary care.

Educational resources

British Thoracic Society: www.brit-thoracic.org.uk
General Practice Airways Group: www.gpiag.org
Asthma UK: www.asthma.org.uk
Scottish Intercollegiate Guidelines Network: www.sign.ac.uk

Resources for patients

Asthma UK provides a useful information base for patients including 'Be in Control' asthma action plan, which can be downloaded direct from their website. Asthma UK also has an interactive demonstration of inhaler technique www.asthma.org.uk/control.

References

British Thoracic Society and Scottish Intercollegiate **Guidelines** Network British guideline on the management of asthma. http://www.brit-thoracic.org.uk/Portals/0/Clinical%20Information/Asthma/Guidelines/asthma_final2008.pdf *Thorax* 2008; 63 (Suppl IV): S1–S121.

Charlton I, Charlton G, Broomfield J, Mullee MA. Audit of the effect of a nurse run asthma clinic on workload and patient morbidity in a general practice. *The British Journal of General Practice* 1991; 41: 227–231.

Clark NM, Gong M, Schork MA et al. Impact of education for physicians on patient outcomes. *Paediatrics* 1998; 101 (5): 831–836.

Dickinson J, Hutton S, Atkin A, Jones K. Reducing asthma morbidity in the community: the effect of a targeted nurse-run asthma clinic in an English general practice. *Respiratory Medicine* 1997; 91 (10): 634–640.

Feder G, Griffiths C, Highton C, Eldridge S, Spena M, Southgate L. Do clinical guidelines introduced with practice based education improve care of asthmatic and diabetic patients? A randomised controlled trial in general practitioners in east London. *British Medical Journal* 1995; 311 (7018): 1473–1478.

Gibson PG & Wilson AJ. The use of continuous quality improvement methods to implement practice guidelines in asthma. *Journal of Quality in Clinical Practice* 1996; 16 (2): 87–102.

Haughney J, Barnes G, Partridge M. Living and breathing: a national survey of patients' views of asthma and its treatment. *Thorax* 2001; 51 (suppl. 3): iii7.

Jones GK, Bell J, Fehrenbach C, Pearce L, Grimley D, McCarthy TP. Understanding patient perceptions of asthma: results of the Asthma Control and Expectations (ACE) survey. *International Journal of Clinical Practice* 2002; 56 (2): 89–93.

Lindberg M, Ahlner J, Moller M, Ekstrom T. Asthma a nurse practice – a resource-effective approach in asthma management. *Respiratory Medicine* 1999; 93 (8): 584–588.

Pinnock H, Bawden R, Proctor S et al. Accessibility, acceptability and effectiveness in primary care of routine telephone review of asthma: pragmatic, randomised controlled trial. *British Medical Journal* 2003; 326 (7387): 477–479.

Premarante UN, Stern JA, Marks GB, Webb JR, Azima H, Burney PG. Clustered randomised trial of an intervention to improve the management of asthma; Greenwich asthma study. *British Medical Journal* 1999; 318 (7193): 1251–1255.

Index

Note: page numbers in *italics* refer to figures, those in **bold** refer to tables and boxes.

CURRENT TITLES

ABC of Skin Cancer

Edited by Sajjad Rajpar & Jerry Marsden
Sandwell & West Birmingham NHS Trust; Selly Oak Hospital, Birmingham

- A new, highly illustrated, concise, factual, and practical overview of skin cancers and pre-cancerous lesions
- Focuses on diagnosis, differential diagnosis, common pitfalls, and outlines best practice management in primary care
- In line with the latest NICE guidelines in the UK, places the emphasis on the pivotal role that GPs play in the screening, diagnosis and referral of skin cancers and pre-cancerous lesions
- Also includes chapters on non-surgical treatment and prevention

April 2008 | 9781405162197 | 80 pages | £19.99/$39.95/€24.90

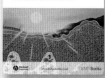

ABC of Clinical Electrocardiography
SECOND EDITION

Edited by Francis Morris, William Brady & John Camm
Northern General Hospital, Sheffield; University of Virginia Health Sciences Centre, Charlottesville; St. George's University of London

- A new edition of this practical guide to the interpretation of ECGs for the non-specialist
- The *ABC* format lends itself to clearly illustrate full 12-lead ECGs
- Sets out the main patterns seen in cardiac disorders in clinical practice, covering the fundamentals of interpretation and analysis
- Covers exercise tolerance testing and provides clear anatomical illustrations to explain key points

May 2008 | 9781405170642 | 112 pages | £26.99/$49.95/€34.90

ABC of Complementary Medicine
SECOND EDITION

Edited by Catherine Zollman, Andrew J. Vickers & Janet Richardson
General Practitioner, Bristol; Memorial Sloan-Kettering Cancer Center, New York; University of Plymouth

- This thoroughly revised and updated second edition offers an authoritative introduction to complementary therapies
- Includes the latest information on efficacy of treatments
- Places a new emphasis in patient management
- Ideal guide for primary care practitioners

June 2008 | 9781405136570 | 64 pages | £21.99/$40.95/€27.90

ABC of Eating Disorders

Edited by Jane Morris
Royal Edinburgh Hospital

- Charts the diagnosis of different eating disorders and their management and treatment by GPs, dieticians and psychiatrists
- Examines diagnosis, management and treatment by health professionals and through self-help
- Helps primary care practitioners recognise eating disorders in young people presenting with other problems
- Supports the work of general psychiatrists and physicians, community health teams and teaching staff
- Includes medico-legal aspects of treating eating disorders and specialist referral

August 2008 | 9780727918437 | 80 pages | £19.99/$35.95/€24.90

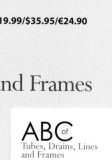

ABC of Tubes, Drains, Lines and Frames

Edited by Adam Brooks, Peter F. Mahoney & Brian Rowlands
Queen's Medical Centre, University of Nottingham; The Royal Centre for Defence Medicine; The Royal Centre for Defence Medicine

- A brand new title in the *ABC* series
- A full-colour, practical guide to the key issues involved in the assessment and management of surgical adjuncts
- Covers the care of post-operative patients in primary care
- Highlights common pitfalls and includes "trouble shooting" sections

October 2008 | 9781405160148 | 88 pages | £19.99/$35.95/€24.90

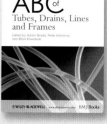

ABC of Headache

Edited by Anne MacGregor & Alison Frith
Both The City of London Migraine Clinic

- Uses real case histories to guide the reader through symptoms to diagnosis and management or, where relevant, to specialist referral
- A highly illustrated, informative and practical source of knowledge and offers links to further information and resources
- An essential guide for healthcare professionals, at all levels of training, looking for possible causes of presenting symptoms of headache

October 2008 | 9781405170666 | 88 pages | £19.99/$35.95/€24.90

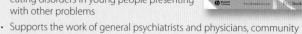

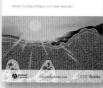

ALSO AVAILABLE

ABC of Adolescence
Russell Viner
2005 | 9780727915740 | 56 pages | £19.99/$35.95/€24.90

ABC of Aids, 5th Edition
Michael W. Adler
2001 | 9780727915030 | 128 pages | £24.99/$46.95/€32.90

ABC of Alcohol, 4th Edition
Alexander Paton & Robin Touquet
2005 | 9780727918147 | 72 pages | £19.99/$35.95/€24.90

ABC of Allergies
Stephen R. Durham
1998 | 9780727912367 | 65 pages | £24.99/$44.95/€32.90

ABC of Antenatal Care, 4th Edition
Geoffrey Chamberlain & Margery Morgan
2002 | 9780727916921 | 92 pages | £22.99/$41.95/€29.90

ABC of Antithrombotic Therapy
Gregory Y.H. Lip & Andrew D. Blann
2003 | 9780727917713 | 67 pages | £19.99/$35.95/€24.90

ABC of Asthma, 5th Edition
John Rees & Dipak Kanabar
2005 | 9780727918604 | 80 pages | £24.99/$44.95/€32.90

ABC of Brainstem Death, 2nd Edition
Christopher Pallis & D.H. Harley
1996 | 9780727902450 | 55 pages | £25.99/$46.95/€32.90

ABC of Breast Diseases, 3rd Edition
J. Michael Dixon
2005 | 9780727918284 | 120 pages | £27.99/$50.95/€34.90

ABC of Burns
Shehan Hettiaratchy, Remo Papini & Peter Dziewulski
2004 | 9780727917874 | 56 pages | £19.99/$35.95/€24.90

ABC of Child Protection, 4th Edition
Sir Roy Meadow, Jacqueline Mok & Donna Rosenberg
2007 | 9780727918178 | 120 pages | £27.99/$50.95/€34.90

ABC of Clinical Genetics, 3rd Edition
Helen M. Kingston
2002 | 9780727916273 | 120 pages | £25.99/$47.95/€32.90

ABC of Clinical Haematology, 3rd Edition
Drew Provan
2007 | 9781405153539 | 112 pages | £27.99/$50.95/€34.90

ABC of Colorectal Cancer
David Kerr, Annie Young & Richard Hobbs
2001 | 9780727915269 | 39 pages | £19.99/$35.95/€24.90

ABC of Colorectal Diseases, 2nd Edition
David Jones
1998 | 9780727911056 | 110 pages | £27.99/$50.95/€34.90

ABC of Conflict and Disaster
Anthony Redmond, Peter F. Mahoney, James Ryan, Cara Macnab & Lord David Owen
2005 | 9780727917263 | 80 pages | £19.99/$35.95/€24.90

ABC of COPD
Graeme P. Currie
2006 | 9781405147118 | 48 pages | £19.99/$35.95/€24.90

ABC of Diabetes, 5th Edition
Peter J. Watkins
2002 | 9780727916938 | 108 pages | £27.99/$50.95/€34.90

ABC of Ear, Nose and Throat, 5th Edition
Harold S. Ludman & Patrick Bradley
2007 | 9781405136563 | 120 pages | £27.99/$50.95/€34.90

ABC of Emergency Radiology, 2nd Edition
Otto Chan
2007 | 9780727915283 | 144 pages | £29.99/$53.95/€37.90

ABC of Eyes, 4th Edition
Peng T. Khaw, Peter Shah & Andrew R. Elkington
2004 | 9780727916594 | 104 pages | £25.99/$46.95/€32.90

ABC of Health Informatics
Frank Sullivan & Jeremy Wyatt
2006 | 9780727918505 | 56 pages | £19.99/$35.95/€24.90

ABC of Heart Failure, 2nd Edition
Russell C. Davis, Michael K. Davies & Gregory Y.H. Lip
2006 | 9780727916440 | 72 pages | £19.99/$35.95/€24.90

ABC of Hypertension, 5th Edition
Gareth Beevers, Gregory Y.H. Lip & Eoin O'Brien
2007 | 9781405130615 | 88 pages | £24.99/$44.95/€32.90

ABC of Intensive Care
Mervyn Singer & Ian Grant
1999 | 9780727914361 | 64 pages | £17.99/$31.95/€24.90

ABC of Interventional Cardiology
Ever D. Grech
2003 | 9780727915467 | 51 pages | £19.99/$35.95/€24.90

ABC of Kidney Disease
David Goldsmith, Satishkumar Abeythunge Jayawardene & Penny Ackland
2007 | 9781405136754 | 96 pages | £26.99/$49.95/€34.90

ABC of Labour Care
Geoffrey Chamberlain, Philip Steer & Luke Zander
1999 | 9780727914156 | 60 pages | £18.99/$33.95/€24.90

ABC of Learning and Teaching in Medicine
Peter Cantillon, Linda Hutchinson & Diana Wood
2003 | 9780727916785 | 64 pages | £18.99/$33.95/€24.90

ABC of Liver, Pancreas and Gall Bladder
Ian Beckingham
2001 | 9780727915313 | 64 pages | £18.99/$33.95/€24.90

ABC of Major Trauma, 3rd Edition
Peter Driscoll, David Skinner & Richard Earlam
1999 | 9780727913784 | 192 pages | £24.99/$46.95/€32.90

ABC of Mental Health
Teifion Davies & T.K.J. Craig
1998 | 9780727912206 | 120 pages | £27.99/$50.95/€34.90

ABC of Monitoring Drug Therapy
Jeffrey Aronson, M. Hardman & D. J. M. Reynolds
1993 | 9780727907912 | 46 pages | £19.99/$35.95/€24.90

ABC of Nutrition, 4th Edition
A. Stewart Truswell
2003 | 9780727916648 | 152 pages | £25.99/$46.95/€32.90

ABC of Obesity
Naveed Sattar & Mike Lean
2007 | 9781405136747 | 64 pages | £19.99/$33.95/€24.90

ABC of Occupational and Environmental Medicine, 2nd Edition
David Snashall & Dipti Patel
2003 | 9780727916112 | 124 pages | £27.99/$50.95/€34.90

ABC of One To Seven, 4th Edition
Bernard Valman
1999 | 9780727912329 | 156 pages | £27.99/$50.95/€34.90

ABC of Oral Health
Crispian Scully
2000 | 9780727915511 | 41 pages | £18.99/$33.95/€24.90

ABC of Palliative Care, 2nd Edition
Marie Fallon & Geoffrey Hanks
2006 | 9781405130790 | 96 pages | £23.99/$44.95/€29.90

ABC of Patient Safety
John Sandars & Gary Cook
2007 | 9781405156929 | 64 pages | £22.99/$40.95/€29.90

ABC of Preterm Birth
William McGuire & Peter Fowlie
2005 | 9780727917638 | 56 pages | £19.99/$35.95/€24.90

ABC of Psychological Medicine
Richard Mayou, Michael Sharpe & Alan Carson
2003 | 9780727915566 | 72 pages | £19.99/$35.95/€24.90

ABC of Resuscitation, 5th Edition
Michael Colquhoun, Anthony Handley & T.R. Evans
2003 | 9780727916693 | 111 pages | £27.99/$50.95/€34.90

ABC of Rheumatology, 3rd Edition
Michael L. Snaith
2004 | 9780727916884 | 136 pages | £25.99/$46.95/€32.90

ABC of Sexual Health, 2nd Edition
John Tomlinson
2004 | 9780727917591 | 96 pages | £24.99/$44.95/€32.90

ABC of Sexually Transmitted Infections, 5th Edition
Michael W. Adler, Frances Cowan, Patrick French, Helen Mitchell & John Richens
2004 | 9780727917614 | 104 pages | £24.99/$46.95/€32.90

ABC of Smoking Cessation
John Britton
2004 | 9780727918185 | 56 pages | £17.99/$33.95/€22.90

ABC of Sports and Exercise Medicine, 3rd Edition
Gregory Whyte, Mark Harries & Clyde Williams
2005 | 9780727918130 | 136 pages | £27.99/$53.95/€34.90

ABC of Subfertility
Peter Braude & Alison Taylor
2004 | 9780727915344 | 64 pages | £18.99/$33.95/€24.90

ABC of the Upper Gastrointestinal Tract
Robert Logan, Adam Harris, J.J. Misiewicz & J.H. Baron
2002 | 9780727912664 | 54 pages | £19.99/$35.95/€24.90

ABC of Urology, 2nd Edition
Chris Dawson & Hugh N. Whitfield
2006 | 9781405139595 | 64 pages | £21.99/$40.95/€27.90

ABC of Wound Healing
Joseph E. Grey & Keith G. Harding
2006 | 9780727916952 | 56 pages | £19.99/$35.95/€24.90

To order call **0800 243407** (UK only) or **+44 1243 843294** (from overseas), email **cs-books@wiley.co.uk** or visit **www.wiley.com**